D0113649

Think Before You Eat

A journey from illness to complete health, taking the reader
step by step to an understanding of the immune system and
information to strengthen it.

Diane Olive

Griffin Publishing
Glendale, California

10   9   8   7   6   5   4   3   2

ISBN 1-882180-25-9

Griffin Publishing
544 Colorado Street
Glendale, California 91204

Telephone: 1-800-423-5789

Manufactured in the United States of America

FOREWORD

Greetings! It was heart-warming to have the chance to provide an introduction for Diane Olive's book *Think Before You Eat*. The statements in this book should be put to practice immediately! I am grateful to Diane for providing this "uncook" book about turning back to nature for fueling the physical and mental self to create a balanced state of mind. I am excited that an increasing number of souls in our society are waking up to the need for a change and are actually getting away from eating addictions which only create more serious problems. I am also encouraged that there are more people in our society opening their minds and hearts to help with the reform. The natural health care alternative is the key because it provides choices and works permanently with very little cost (except discipline), and provides the control through eating habits. This change requires that we be responsible for our physical and mental well-being. Naturally, we have great benefits in store as we reveal, reconnect, and rejuvenate to wellness and provide the body and mind with self-healing. I am happy that Diane is providing this very fine book *Think before You Eat*. When reading it I found treasures of information from the many weeks, hours, and months she spent preparing this book. I appreciate the time that Diane has taken to provide such a wide variety of information. The scientific data from the research on the values of food was indeed a great contribution.

With blessing for good reading that is going to be a very great help to you.

Ann Wigmore

DISCLAIMER

The opinions expressed in this book are solely the author's and are based on the extensive research that she has conducted. The author does not directly or indirectly dispense medical advice or prescribe the information contained in this book as a form of treatment for any physical or mental ailment without medical approval. Anyone seeking medical advice should contact a qualified licensed health practitioner. The intent is to offer information that may help you and your chosen health practitioner work better together in your mutual quest for health.

CONTENTS

ACKNOWLEDGMENTS

Thanks to my parents Donna and Herman Rosenthal, Dean Black, Mr. and Mrs. Eugene Briggs, Dr. Tei Fu Chen, Charlotte Gerson, the Natural Hygiene Society, Ann Wigmore and all the people who helped me learn about health.

PERMISSIONS

American Natural hygiene Society, Inc, 11816 Pace Track Rd, Tampa Fl 33626.

Herbert Shelton, "Fasting Can Save Your Life," *Junior Hygienist*, 3 paragraphs: para 4,5, p. 71 para 1, p. 72.

For more information on the original studies conducted by Francis M Pottenger, Jr, M.D., please contact the: Price-Pottenger Nutrition Foundation, P.O. 2614 La Mesa, CA. 91943-2614/ (619)574-7763.

Table of food Composition provided by Elizabeth Baker/ Drewlwood Communications.

Foot Reflexology Chart form "Foot Notes: A step-by-step guide to the practice of Foot Reflexology" by Sr. Mary Em McGlone, 8400 Pine Rd Philadelphia PA 19111.

Food Combining Chart, Shangri-La Health Resort.

Paramid Energy, Mary Hardy.

Colette Coglandro.

SW. Nostradamus Virato, founder & executive editor, *New Frontier Magazine*.

Raw Foods, Susan Jorg.

INTRODUCTION

At the age of twenty-three I became seriously ill, going again and again to many physicians for help. They tried but never did get to the cause of my problems. Each doctor proclaimed different medical diagnoses—allergies, irritable bowel syndrome, parasites, a too narrow urethra, and finally, 'its all in your head'. Their remedies were the same drugs. I followed their advice and took the drugs. But at the age of thirty, I found that my condition had worsened. I had developed intense environmental allergies, arthritis, ulcers, problems with walking, and unrelenting pain in my body. After seven years of this treatment, I knew the doctors alone couldn't help me. I had to take responsibility for my health to begin searching for the cause of my suffering.

My search led me to bookstores, libraries, health food stores, Natural Hygiene Philosophy, Chinese medicine, holistic health doctors, and alternative (to the MD's) therapies. My conclusion was that my body had taken in too many toxins (antibiotics, paints, mercury) and not enough clean raw whole food.

I learned and started applying some incredibly simple principles to my life. Namely, maintain a positive mental attitude, and get lots of restful sleep, exercise, pure water and sunshine. Eat clean whole food grains, herbs, fruits, nuts, seeds, and vegetables. And make a conscious effort to bring my body into balance. By following the principles, I became the healthiest and happiest I have ever been.

This book is written to help others understand how things we do affect us and our neighbors. I discuss many subjects energy exchange, enzymes, dental (mercury amalgams) fillings, toxins, protein, food combining, five senses, doctors, children, Chinese health philosophy, Dr. Dean Black, menstrual periods, old age, the future, and food recipes.

Each of us is responsible to create balance in our bodies and balance in our community and world. An excellent way to begin improving our balance is to improve our diet. When we eat toxic, dead, or poor quality food, we confuse our body's energy flow and eventually we malfunction. Observe the imbalance energy flow (behavior) that a large percentage of us have. We are too aggressive (too Yang—yelling, stealing, sickly, fighting, being disagreeable) or too passive (too Yin—dull, weak, lazy, overweight, sick). I believe that changing to a diet that is naturally correct can help correct out of balance energy flows in our bodies. I learned too that mother nature (earth) has its own heart beat (rhythms) as obviously manifested in tides and seasons. Perhaps, listening to mother nature and getting in balance with her flow of life, eating her foods, seeing her beauty, filling her and our mutual needs, using (not interfering with) what she provides only this can return peace and paradise to the world!

1

THE UNFORGETTABLE SCENE

The bald-headed doctor leaned forward in his chair putting his face uncomfortably close to mine. His warm moist breath engulfed my tear-covered face. His small eyes peered over his spectacles. He stared at me, as if I were a child needing direction. Calmly and clearly he pronounced, "You must go and see a psychiatrist." As he spoke, the pain rose from my feet and legs to penetrate my body. I cried silently— "Why won't you help me? Please, make the pain go away." He insisted that he couldn't help because my problems were psychological. This didn't satisfy me. I wanted a better answer. The idea of it all being inside my head was laughable. What about my allergy to gluten and dairy products, the terrible pains in my body, my indigestion, insomnia and spastic colon? These problems were in my body not in my head! Why was I, at the age of twenty-nine, suffering all this?

If you looked at me you would never know that anything was wrong. I looked normal. I was 5'6", weighed 110 pounds, had long thick dark brown curly hair and large green eyes. The doctor did not understand the severe pain I was enduring.

This wise and powerful doctor's confident diagnosis happened within the first hour of meeting me. The embarrassment from being told this in front of my husband, John, was indescribable. He turned to John and said, "Take her to the best qualified psychiatrist. I am sure this is the problem. Bring back the results." This was the diagnosis of a specialist in allergies. On our way home, John said, "Why don't we go and see a psychiatrist?" My dear husband, my best friend, agreed with the doctor. I was in total shock. I yelled, "There's nothing wrong with my mind, so there must be something wrong with everyone else!" I cried until my eyes were swollen, my face beet red.

When we reached home in Philadelphia, I rushed inside and telephoned my father at his work-place in San Diego. I told him what happened and how terrible I felt. I asked him if he thought the doctor was right. He replied, "No, Diane, you are not crazy. There is something wrong with your body, not your mind." Thank goodness. Someone believed me.

This scene is so unforgettable it caused me to write this book. In the following pages, I will share with you my journey from the horrible state of unrelenting pain, increasing sickness, and deep depression to the joy of wonderful health and a better understanding of life.

By nature I am a fighter. When given a challenge I grab it, try to understand why it came about, and look for the wisdom to solve it. For example, an unusually strong challenge faced me several years ago while studying art at San Diego State University. I had been painting for twelve years, having decided since age five that I had to be an artist. I felt that the teachers were not helping me to express myself and that I was not learning the things that I should. I thought about what was needed to solve this limitation. I listed on paper the negatives and positives for the situation. The negatives outweighed the positive; therefore, at the age of twenty-three, I changed schools to California State Northridge in Los Angeles. The change was good because the Art teachers in Los Angeles allowed me the freedom to communicate my ideas and to express myself through my own choice of color and line. Here, Art was what I thought it should be. These teachers warned me that everything in Art had already been done—there were no new ideas left. This seemed so odd that I filed the comment away. Even though I did not agree with it, I always was open to new views. I enjoyed my new school tremendously. Almost all the Art teachers were exhibiting their work in galleries. Art and my fiancee, John, were my only cares in the world.

John was a former professional basketball player, 6'7", 220 pounds, 27 years old, with dark Italian features. So nice, that sometimes I was envious of his courteous ways, hoping that his kindness and good manners would rub off on me.

John enjoyed taking me out to dinner. Our favorite activity was to travel one hour south from beautiful San Diego, down the rocky Pacific coast to the town of Newport, Mexico. There we'd drive along the beach on bright sunny sleepy afternoons, enjoying the foods and sights of Mexico. We dined on piping-hot, buttery lobster, wonderfully served with steaming corn tortillas, rice, and creamy beans. We usually washed this food down with Mexico's finest, bubbly Corona beer, to get that relaxed state with which to enjoy the sunshine. Unfortunately, I also got sick when I ate these foods, often coming down with diarrhea from these fine tasty meals. I was having so much fun that I never even gave much thought to this problem. I just assumed it was an inevitable part of traveling.

Immediately after returning from these trips, I would check in with the knowledgeable school doctor and ask him for relief. He always diagnosed a parasite and prescribed a cure-all antibiotic. I followed directions, swallowed the magic drug for ten days, and miraculously my diarrhea vanished, or so I thought.

A dramatic increase of this problem seemed to happen overnight when I was twenty-three years old. One morning I woke up not only with diarrhea but with an added complication, a bladder infection (E. Coli). Now the prescription said "Take the antibiotics for two months." I did and my bladder quit hurting, but when I stopped swallowing the pills my bladder became sore again. What to do now? Of course, repeat the cycle of pill taking again for two more months. The results—same as before. Since I was not improving, I sought a new doctor, this time an expert—a Urologist. He examined me, decided my urethra was not wide enough, stretched it in a hospital and promised that this procedure would prevent future infection. No luck. My bladder remained sore, the diarrhea continued. So back to another expert doctor I went.

This time, to a Gastroenterologist, to get his solution. He decided that I had Inflammatory Bowel Disease. For relief certain foods must be eliminated from my diet. He said milk lactose cannot be digested without proper digestive enzymes and I was missing those enzymes. But don't worry! This wasn't unusual. Many people had this disorder. Also, he said that when I ate vegetables they would irritate my digestive system and cause my intestines to stay sore. His solution—

don't drink milk and don't eat raw vegetables—seemed reasonable, so I quit eating them.

The doctor said there is no cure for irritable bowels—you just have to live with it. I felt a little better not eating raw foods and dairy products, but I still knew there was something wrong with my body. Many others suffered with and accepted this disorder. Well, then I must accept it and the pain that accompanied it. John felt it wasn't so horrible and there were people with a lot worse problems. That was true—so live with it I did.

What primed me for such horrible degeneration? It could have been my night manicurist job in a beauty salon during the school year. The job required applying nail polish and attaching acrylic nails to a person's own fingernails. The false nail was bonded by means of a catalyst so powerful I always became dizzy applying it. I discovered later that the formaldehyde in the nail polish is the same stuff used to embalm dead bodies. Daily I breathed the potent fumes from hair dyes, hair spray and other chemicals floating throughout the beauty salon. There was no escaping chemicals even at school. The school required a full eight hours a day, five to six days a week, in an atmosphere that constantly exposed the students to harmful oil paints containing heavy metals such as lead, chromium, etc. There were no warning labels (this was to come seven years later). I didn't even think about the health hazards since I was used to having these paints on my hands and lips since I was ten years old. Turpentine, with its fantastic aroma, still evokes in me the memories of studios, paints, and Art. Never once did I think about the large danger sign on the turpentine can.

And how about my diet? Even though it was better than the standard American junk food diet, I gave it no real thought. I had no time for food. Breakfast was granola or eggs. It was health food granola, of course, with lots of cooked honey and roasted oats—just keep the belly full and on we go.

Lunch was a quick tuna sandwich, dripping in mayonnaise and enclosed in air-whipped, bleached white bread, fortified with vitamins originally removed when the flour was processed. Yes, red tomato and a bit of lettuce were added for color.

Dinner usually was fish or chicken with cooked vegetables such as broccoli, carrots, potatoes or corn. I was determined not to irritate my colon with anything raw like a salad and avoided fruit because this might contribute to the problem.

Everybody took vitamin pills since this was how you obtained your needed nutrients. It's not necessary to eat good food. Just make up the inadequacies in poor food by supplementing them with vitamin pills. Isn't this what we learned in nutrition class in school? I had that famous "one" class which informed us as to what we needed to sustain life and thought I understood! I still remember the acronym RDA. Normal recommended daily allowances (RDA's) of vitamin and minerals are set by the Food and Nutrition Board of the National Academy of Sciences, National Research Council. They periodically update their recommendations, which are "designed for the maintenance of good nutrition of practically all healthy people in the US"

Why worry about diet? I didn't need to understand the value of a good diet. Experts had already studied it. I wasn't an expert. I was taught to follow their recommendations.

Unfortunately, even though I followed the expert advice, I didn't get better. So every year I went back to different doctors. The doctors at Scripps Clinic in San Diego ran blood tests. They found nothing. It was the same old story—I would just have to live with my problems. Once in a while they would give me more antibiotics to see if it was a reoccurrence of a parasite. But, no such luck.

In 1986 I married and moved to Philadelphia. My husband was hired as an assistant basketball coach for Villanova University. We were excited about his opportunity and quickly accepted the position. I was madly in love with my husband and would follow him anywhere.

I was lucky and became pregnant on my honeymoon. We were ecstatic about having a baby. I bought every book I could find on the subject of birth. My first thing each morning was to read the books and study the pictures of the growing fetus. The science of childbirth was truly remarkable! Morning sickness was to be expected for three months; however, my "morning sickness" occurred at night.

I was working as a children's art teacher, but in my sixth month I couldn't continue because of pains in my back. So what—I was having a baby! It was an honor to be a woman and to be able to grow a living being in my belly.

Three months later my baby was on its way. My contractions lasted for three days and two sleepless nights with pain that was unbearable! On May 18, 1986, I had a natural delivery, in the hospital, of a beautiful and healthy baby girl whom we named Jacklyn Rose.

Having Jacklyn did not keep my health from becoming worse. I became nervous about breast feeding because of my increasing food allergies. Gluten was now greatly feared (gluten is in wheat flour, oats, barley and rye). At first I didn't know that these grains were loaded with gluten. But I learned the truth fast because whenever I ate one of them my bowels would go into spasms.

What exactly is gluten? Well, if you take a spoonful of wheat flour and mix it with a little water the result will be a pliable sort of paste, firmly bonded together. The ingredient that makes it bind like this is gluten, says Rita Greer, in her book *Gluten-Free Cooking*. Gluten is so strong that before modern adhesives were developed, it was used as a paste to glue wallpaper onto walls.

When one has a weak digestive system, they are not able to break down the gluten; therefore, it may deposit as a sticky coating on the villi of their intestines. The normal function of the villi is to soak in food and absorb nutrients, but when coated with gluten the villi can't perform their intended function. Doctors and medical literature say there is no cure for a person with gluten intolerance.

Gluten intolerance, also called Sprue or Celiac Disease, is characterized by sore mouth and tongue, anemia, severe diarrhea, and large amounts of fats in stools. Resulting gas distention and pain in the abdomen are usually acute and stools often contain so much gas that they are frothy. The tiny finger-like villi that normally cover the walls of the small intestines also become shortened, fuse together, or may be absent, thus decreasing the absorption of nutrients to only a fraction of that of a healthy individual.

This disease can be life threatening and before gluten-free diets were used, a large percentage of children with Celiac disease died. Mild symptoms of this disease have been produced in volunteers who ate large amounts (100 grams) of gluten daily for ten weeks.[1]

---

[1] Rita Greer, *Gluten-Free Cooking*, p.7.

I quit eating gluten and felt better. Doing this limited my choice of foods, making it difficult for me to eat in restaurants. I switched my starch intake to corn, rice, sweet potato, and white potato.

My family and career took a back burner to this great burden of ill-health. The fear of not knowing what was wrong with me was draining. Except for my family (my mother and father continued to try to help me), I was alone in my search.

My mother's research concluded that my problems were caused by antibiotics. She said I had taken too many antibiotics and had upset the balance between friendly and unfriendly intestinal flora in my body. She felt this caused an overgrowth of unfriendly bacteria called Candida Albicans, or sometimes simply called Yeast, which was destroying my body. I knew I had vaginal yeast infections in the past, but my doctors never said it was also growing in my intestines. For six years I had noticed that my stools had been coated with mucus but I didn't know what that meant; fortunately, my mother did and she mailed me books and articles on Candida so that I could understand what was happening.

2

CANDIDA

WHAT IS CANDIDA ALBICANS?

Candida Albicans is a yeast growing in all of us, and is normally controlled by good bacteria in the intestines. But, when something destroys the helpful bacteria, the yeast begins to invade and colonize the body tissue. These yeast colonies can release powerful chemicals into the bloodstream, to cause such varying symptoms as lethargy, chronic diarrhea, constipation, yeast vaginitis, bladder infections, menstrual cramps, asthma, migraine headaches, and severe depression.[1]

William G. Crook, MD, author of *The Yeast Connection*, and Sidney Baker, MD, lay much of the actual increase of Candidiasis, the overgrowth of Candida Albicans, to their own profession who may be overusing antibiotics. They consider that the misuse of antibiotics is a legacy of the era of the 1940's and 1950's when "play it safe" doctors routinely prescribed them for patients with sore throats and fevers.

I asked a pharmacist who worked in a hospital what she knew about Candida Albicans. She said, "Candida is the bacteria that takes over the body when you are dying. You usually only see this in the hospitals when the patient is dying or has been given too many drugs."

Candida Albicans is a very serious disease if allowed to thrive and be left untreated. It now may be as common as premenstrual syndrome. In fact, the two diseases may go hand-in-hand. Many of the symptoms in both conditions are considered unimportant by doctors, so they go untreated and

---

[1] Louise Tenney, *Candida Albicans.*

undiagnosed. One woman I interviewed was told by her doctor that she had mental problems, and that it was all in her head. Sound familiar?

How can you tell if you have excessive yeast? There is no way of telling by a lab test. Since the yeast naturally occurs in our bodies, who is to say how much is excessive enough to bother the patient? Glamour magazine reports: "Since yeast is present in everyone, its presence in lab tests does not necessarily confirm that growth is out of hand. The most effective test is trial or treatment, through change in diet and an antibacterial drug or herb."

Another article advises patients to stop using antibiotics long-term and to use other forms of birth control than the pill. They insist that foods containing sugar be eliminated from the diet.

This recommended common diet was also printed in *Redbook*, April 1986, under the heading, "THE NEWEST MYSTERY ILLNESS."

THE ANTI-YEAST DIET

REFINED CARBOHYDRATES. Avoid sugar, white flour, white rice.

SUGAR-CONTAINING FOODS AND BEVERAGES. Also, do not use maple syrup, molasses, honey.

YEAST AND FOODS CONTAINING YEAST. These include yeast breads, rolls, crackers and snack foods containing yeast; natural vitamins with yeast in them; brewer's or nutritional yeast. *Read labels carefully.*

ALCOHOLIC BEVERAGES. Liquor, beer, wine and cider are taboo. All are made with yeast.

CHEESE. The more aged a cheese, the more yeast it contains. Some doctors allow cream cheese, cottage cheese and ricotta.

PRODUCTS OF YEAST FERMENTATION. This category includes all vinegars and products containing vinegar (pickles, mayonnaise, catsup, many salad dressings, barbecue sauce, etc.), soy sauce, sour cream and buttermilk. Sugar-free, fruit-free yogurt is usually allowed—it is fermented with the friendly bacteria lactobacillus, not yeast.

PROCESSED FOODS. These are apt to contain more yeast than non-processed foods. Avoid bacon, ham lox, beef jerky and other smoked meats and fish, as well as dried fruits and dried vegetables. Some doctors even prohibit dried herbs, including teas.

FRUITS AND FRUIT JUICES. Fruits are quickly converted by the body into sugar. And some fruits, especially cantaloupe and other melons, may be contaminated with mold. Canned and bottled fruit juices are loaded with yeast. After several weeks, if you find you're improving, you can try having freshly squeezed orange juice or whole fruits to see if they provoke symptoms.

COFFEE AND TEA. These are subject to mold contamination, although how much is uncertain. If you feel you can't get along without these beverages, try cutting down and observing your reactions.

FOOD ADDITIVES: Many doctors prohibit foods and beverages with artificial flavors, colors and preservatives.

FOODS ALLOWED: All vegetables; eggs; whole grains such as rice, wheat, oats, barley and millet; chicken, fish, seafood and lean meats; butter and unprocessed vegetable oils.

The Candida books and articles suggest a diet high in protein and low in fruit. Note that to prevent cancer, the American Cancer Society was saying just the opposite—diets low in protein and high in fruits (and vegetables). This Candida diet didn't make sense to me, but I wanted to get better and I tried it.

Finally, anti-fungal drugs such as Nystatin are prescribed to suppress the growth of the yeast. Caprylic acid, garlic, Pau D'Arco, and vitamins are also recommended. I tried them all and had awful die-offs. What are die-offs?

There were large warning signs as the books and magazines talked about killing the yeast, causing die-offs. In *The Yeast Connection,* William Crook, MD, writes, "Die-off: when you kill the yeast germs in your intestinal, respiratory or vaginal membranes you absorb products from these dead yeast germs which temporarily worsen your symptoms...Each person is different. Die-off symptoms include fatigue, depression, aching and feeling slowed down and cold."

I took my Candida books to my disease specialist HMO doctors. They said that there was no such thing as Candida disease. The books and articles I had on Candida were not true. But, I told them, "Doctors just like yourself wrote those Candida books." Their attitude completely confused me, leaving me not knowing who to believe. My list of illnesses was looked upon as just complaints. They laughed at the profusion of illnesses in the books saying "They are trying to say all illness stems from Candida—which can't be true."

They told me to go see a doctor of gastroenterology. I did. The specialist in Gastroenterology and Internal Medicine didn't believe in Candida either. He decided to do an upper and lower GI, a colonoscopy and look directly into my bowel and stomach. I will never forget the pain of the colonoscopy. It was worse than having a baby. The doctor took a snake-like, long black tube with a light on the end and inserted it all the way through my colon, inch by inch, scream by scream. I never yelled once while having my baby, so I am not a wimp. After inspecting my lower colon, the doctor said, "Your colon looks fine," and then suggested medication to calm down the spastic colon. I had just been through the worst pain in my life only to be told there were no answers once again.

One thing he did suggest was Metamucil. I did not understand why he wanted me to take fiber. Wasn't fiber the thing I should avoid? I bought the Metamucil but never took it, putting it on the shelf to gather dust. At the time I thought it had to be the last thing I needed. Too bad the doctor didn't explain how fiber worked. It is so simple—fiber is like a broom sweeping the colon clean. He didn't even suggest a book for me to read, he didn't take the time. Also, he could have evaluated my diet. He did tell me to go to a dietitian. I went to the dietitian. She told me not to visit the health food store anymore. She said, "They're all nuts. There is no such thing as Candida. Stay on your gluten-free diet, but eat at least one salad a week. Wine is fine once in a while." I tried her diet, drank one glass of wine and became worse. This isn't surprising to me now because people with Candida imbalances already have a yeast problem in their bodies, so why feed them more yeast products?

I was trying hard to believe in the conventional medical doctors, but this only caused more pain and conflicting solutions. The last HMO doctor I visited was the allergist who decided I needed a psychiatrist. This was the last straw; no more HMO doctors for me. The HMO health insurance was costing us one hundred dollars a month for these "free" visits. I didn't want the uninformed specialist advice anymore, so I called our insurance company and asked if they had any doctors in their plan who specialized in Candida. They didn't. I now understood, except for my family, I was alone. I had to take responsibility for my health. There did not appear to be any professional who would help me. I realized that health care isn't free. My money and my time were no longer going to be given to these uncaring specialists. I would take my money and search for the answer my way.

The first place I went to was the "forbidden" health food store to get their recommendations on Candida doctors. I telephoned each doctor, ensuring they had researched Candida disease.

I discussed this with my husband who told me he was against seeing a doctor who specialized in Candida. He felt we were going to the outer edge of the medical profession: any doctor who specialized in something that did not exist was probably a quack. He said that we must stay in the borders of the traditional medical doctors and that seeing a psychiatrist was a better idea. Needless to say, we had a terrible argument.

I was going to a Candida doctor, whether he liked it or not. Reluctantly, and because he loved me, John went with me to see the Candida specialist. Interestingly, this doctor was the only doctor to have sympathy for my problems. He told me his story. He had suffered a similar problem, Crohn's Disease. His doctors wanted to remove a section of his bowel, but not wanting to destroy his body he refused to agree to this. Rather, he decided to try to improve his health through diet. He was somewhat successful and became better through diet changes and vitamin supplements. Most of his knowledge was obtained through self experimentation. He had tried Nystatin, becoming very sick with the die-offs. He learned to be careful with doses of it and with the other helpful substances such as Pau D'Arco, Caprylic Acid, rutin and garlic. They all destroyed the Candida, but in doing so released toxins to circulate in the blood. This caused him to suffer severe reactions.

He put me on megadoses of isolated vitamins and the traditional Candida diet: low fruit, low starch, four ounces or less, gluten-free, no dairy, high protein, and lots of vegetables. I also had to avoid the night shade plants (white potato, tomatoes, green, red and black pepper and eggplant) which could cause joint pain, insomnia, and arthritis.

In *Potatoes* by Alvin and Virginia B. Silverstein, I learned, "As knowledge of botany increased...it was realized that potatoes are a member of the nightshade family, many of whose members produce deadly poisons...The leaves and stems of a potato plant look very much like those of tomatoes. This is no coincidence as many members of this family have a sinister reputation, for they produce poisonous alkaloids such as the drug belladonna." In the article, "Boning up on Osteoporosis," Mark Mead writes, "Also problematic are the nightshade vegetables, such as tomatoes and eggplant, which contain certain acids that interfere with calcium use."

Not eating nightshades helped me tremendously. The pains in my feet and legs as well as the insomnia disappeared in two weeks. However, if afterwards, I ate even a small piece of potato, I paid for it terribly, suffering with intense pain. It could take up to a week to get the nightshades out of my system and the pains out of my body.

I felt so much better on this diet and was on the road to recovery. Within two weeks I was walking a mile a day. We started talking about having another baby. This was it! I finally found a doctor who knew how to help me.

3

MERCURY AMALGAMS

One subject the Candida doctor and I discussed was his concern about my dental fillings. These fillings are fifty-percent mercury, maybe one of the deadliest poisons known to mankind. Dentists currently are divided as to how to advise their patients; divided because in most cases, the manifestations of mercury poisoning may not start to become apparent until three to ten years after the insertion of the mercury.

"Scientific research has demonstrated that mercury, even in small amounts, can damage the brain, heart, lungs, liver, kidneys, thyroid gland, pituitary gland, adrenal glands, blood cells, enzymes, hormones, and suppresses the body's immune (defense) system. In addition, mercury has been shown to pass through the placental membrane of pregnant women and cause permanent damage to the brain of a developing baby."[1]

If it can pass through the placenta, what about breast milk? Cherill Miles of Nebraska gave birth in a hospital to a healthy baby boy named Mark. The first two nights in the hospital the baby was fine. Once Cherill's breast milk came in the baby became fussy, refusing her milk. Cherill pumped her breast milk and gave it to Mark, but he still did not want the milk. Because of the sucking reflex she force fed him while sleeping.

> Many times I just dumped my milk down the sink. I also noticed a metallic odor to the milk. He developed dark circles under his eyes, and bad breath. The doctor said, 'he is the youngest baby I have ever seen develop shingles.' A red rash covered his entire face. I had to use a suppository every time to get his bowels moving. He only slept for fifteen minutes at a time—then woke up crying. Mark

[1] C. Ray Kaiser, AA, BA, MA, *The Par Booklet*, p.28.

would be up all night long crying, he cried for four days straight. I had no sleep and became irritable and begged God to take one of us—it didn't matter anymore, because I just couldn't take the crying. I went from doctor to doctor and no one knew how to help me. Mark was ten months old when I found a homeopathic doctor. He ran tests on the baby and said we were mercury toxic. He said to stop breast feeding Mark immediately. When I gave the baby formula, he drank it like crazy and just could not get enough—he stopped crying, started sleeping through the night, and moved his bowels on his own two or three times a day.

When Cherill was eighteen years old her dentist had put the first silver fillings into her mouth—fourteen of them. Right after this she developed constipation, only going once every seven to fourteen days. She also developed other symptoms—depression, fatigue and irritability.

The Candida doctor said it would be okay to have my fillings removed. However, he told me that he had his taken out and felt no difference. I decided I needed more concrete evidence before I would have mine removed, so I started researching the subject.

Mercury is one of the oldest recognized and strongest poisons known. And yet, Dentists have placed amalgam fillings (commonly used ones average 52% pure mercury) in our teeth for over 150 years. Why would they do this if the material is poisonous?

"When amalgam was originally introduced in the United States around 1830, the then National Dental Association sternly warned against its use. The alternative material at that time, however, was gold; and amalgam was a cheaper, easier-to-use alternative; therefore, it gained popular acceptance in the dental profession."[1]

Cheaper and easier was the answer then, but now there is no excuse. There is a large selection of alternative materials which can restore up to 98% of the original tooth.

From 1900 to 1970, the dentist mixed his own metal powders to form fillings, but now it is known to be far too dangerous to be handling these metal powders. The American Dental Association (ADA) now delivers the mercury filling capsules already premixed to be put in the mouth.

---

[1] Sam Ziff and Michael F. Ziff, *The Hazards of Silver/Mercury Dental Fillings*, pp. 1, 7, 19.

I asked a dentist friend of ours if there was any truth to the fillings being toxic. He immediately said, "Absolutely not—the fillings release no mercury at all. This is what we were taught in Dental School and by the ADA." He wrote to the American Dental Association to get their position. The ADA sent him an envelope filled with information on their opinion, including a statement of the Council On Ethics of the ADA and *The Use of Mercury in Dentistry*; also, a critical review of recent literature written by Dan C. Langen, DDS, PL, PhD and Alice A. Hoos was enclosed.

After reading the studies he said that mercury does leak out of the fillings, but in such "safe" small amounts that it shouldn't bother anyone. Also, he realized he would be termed a quack by his colleagues and the ADA if he were to start replacing mercury fillings.

The major problem stressed in the article, "The Use of Mercury in Dentistry," was not the effects on the patient, but concern for mercury poisoning of the dentist. The dentists were careless in the care of the amalgams.

Now, a "no touch" technique under the following guidelines should be used for handling amalgams.

1. Expressing excess mercury from amalgams should be avoided.

2. Amalgamator arms and capsules should be covered.

3. Scrap amalgams should be stored in sealed containers.

4. Amalgams should be stored away from heat.

5. Amalgam contaminated instruments should be thoroughly cleaned before sterilization.

6. Disposable items contaminated with mercury should be discarded in properly sealed containers.

7. During removal of amalgam restorations, the use of a water spray and high volume evacuation greatly reduces mercury vapor levels.

8. Good ventilation with rapid fresh air exchange and an outside exhaust is extremely important to prevent inhalation of mercury vapor.

Also, mercury spills may lodge in carpeting and cracks in the floor. This is where they think the problem lies—not in one's mouth. Mercury can be in the mouth for ages with no concern from the ADA or the Safety and Health Organization. Personally, I don't think it makes any sense to embed a poison in your mouth, because then you are exposed to the deadly poisonous mercury twenty-four hours a day, every day of the week. Think about it. Each time you chew or brush your teeth you are likely to erode off the mercury and release its vapors into your body. But, the ADA implies, no problem. It is in small safe amounts.

Let's take a closer look at their own tests reported in a review article. Measurable amounts of mercury vapor have been found in the expired air of patients with amalgam restorations. In addition, increases in the amount of mercury vapor were observed after chewing and brushing.

A study to measure mercury concentration was conducted using 80 subjects—40 with amalgams and 40 without. Mercury concentrations were measured by collecting 2.7 liters of expired air in a plastic bag and passing it through a gold foil mercury vapor analyzer. At the start of the experiment, a sample was taken "at rest" before chewing. Even at this stage, those with the amalgams showed three (3) times more mercury exposure at 0.88μg/cu m then those without, whose exposure was 0.26μg/cu m.

After vigorous chewing for 10 minutes, the mercury concentration was 0.13μg/cu m for the amalgamless group and 13.74μg/cu m for the amalgam group."[1] Note that the amalgam group produces one hundred times the amount of the other group. Could this be a dangerous exposure?

Metal fillings are like having a battery run through your body. If you put on too many lights or electricity you short circuit the house—the same with your body.

A simple "NO" to mercury amalgams before they are put in your mouth should do the trick. You may say, "None of this is true. The ADA, the government and health organizations are looking out for me. They care about me! If they say mercury is safe in my mouth, then it is safe." Are you sure that a lot of people care about you? Consider the pesticides in our food and water, and air pollution. And how about this for a shocker. It only took one person to blow the whistle on the trucks hauling waste one way, but carrying food products on the return trip in the same vehicle.

[1] Dan C. Langon, DDS, PL Fan, PhD, and Alice A. Hoos, *JADA Review*, "The Use of Mercury in Dentistry, a critical review of the recent literature," p. 21.

I thought that it would be a good idea to have the waste (amalgams) in my mouth removed by my dentist in Philadelphia. To make sure I was making the right decision, I first took tests as described by The Center, a center created by a dentist. At my request the Center sent my dentist their amalgam removal procedures and recommended tests for detecting mercury or metal poisoning in hair, urine, and blood. My dentist gave me the tests and found that I had a large amount of mercury in my body. I decided to have my amalgams replaced with composite materials provided that he would follow the Center's procedures. Being very cautious, I knew that I must pay strict attention to the dentists and others who have warned that amalgam removal can be dangerous if proper procedures are not followed.

"We get numerous phone calls each day from patients who have either accidentally or intentionally omitted the steps in proper amalgam removal (PAR). These patients report a variety of resulting complications. Some have gone into shock, some have shown premature ventricular contraction, some have been hospitalized, and some have been placed in mental institutions."[1]

I went through the PAR steps as the experts suggested. It cost (for tests and vitamin supplements) roughly $1,000 and on May 25, 1988, I had three fillings out of my thirteen removed. First, my dentist sealed off the back of my throat with a rubber dam to ensure that the pieces of the amalgams would not fall down my throat while he drilled. Then he injected Novocain into my mouth. The sharp needle stung me like a wild mosquito over and over until it reached its numbing goal. A loud buzzing noise of the drill made me feel stiff and frightened as if I were a building under construction. The dentist said sternly, "Relax, you're too nervous."

I observed the metal dust flying thickly in the air. A young female dental hygienist used an instrument to vacuum up the toxic dust while the dentist drilled on. Once she forgot to use the suction and I breathed in a cloud of dangerous metal particles.

After two very long hours, the three fillings were removed. Now I could get up, walk out the door and never come back. I

---

[1] Sam Ziff and Michael F. Ziff, *The Hazards of Silver/Mercury Dental Fillings*, p. 19.

decided in that dental chair that I didn't care how many fillings needed to be replaced. It was far worse having them removed than leaving them in my mouth. But, as I tried to get up from the chair, I found that I had no strength. It was a hard effort for me. I finally stood up even though my body was trembling and my heart was racing. I felt exhausted and started going into spasms of crying. What had happened? I didn't know why, but I could not stop myself from crying. After ten minutes of my shaking, the dentist looked at me caringly and said, "It's all the tension and anxiety of having the fillings removed." (Once again the medical diagnosis was that my emotions were causing the problem. In other words, I was inflicting this misery on myself.) Immediately, I called my husband and told him to come and pick me up. I was a mess and not in any condition to drive myself home.

I went home that day to start a living hell that no one should ever have to experience. All night long my heart kept racing. John could feel my strong heart beat and racing pulse. I could not sleep that night or the next. Weeks would go by without any normal sleep. A burning pain brushed over the tops of my legs and across my back, as if someone was holding a hot flame close to my skin. My stomach stopped working, allowing food to be left undigested in my bowels.

I called the "Candida doctor" to ask him what was happening to me. He thought that I could be allergic to the Novocain or that I could be suffering from mercury poisoning. He advised me to take more glutathione and Vitamin C to help get rid of the poisons. Taking them caused me to have even more burning on the tops of my legs and on the inside lining of my stomach.

Feeling worse, I called the Dentist's Diagnostic Center for more help. A female nutritional consultant answered the telephone and quietly said, "Yes, we have been getting many phone calls this month from patients complaining of digestive upsets and stomach burning after going through The Center's procedures. I don't know how to help you or the others. Maybe you could try our brand of Vitamin C, vitamins, and charcoal."

I was furious. I followed all the PAR steps. This was not supposed to happen. I followed the rules, but still I suffered from the frying pan syndrome. I didn't realize how dangerous the amalgams were. Instead of releasing mercury slowly over the years, the removal of three fillings at one time had shocked my immune system AND NEARLY KILLED ME.

My digestion was a mess. The food stuck in my stomach and rotted. I kept burping up a smelly, rotten, bad-tasting odor. Irritation of my stomach lining grew more intense as the weeks went on, finally causing me pain even when I drank water.

Tearfully I called the doctor every day. I asked him how and what I should be eating to lessen the stomach pain. Vegetables irritated my stomach more than white rice and chicken. He told me to take out the vegetables and eat every two hours to keep my stomach coated with food. "Isn't it dangerous not to eat vegetables? I asked the doctor. He answered, "No, it's fine for a few months—bland food calms the stomach."

I went to the library to research the medical books on ulcerated stomachs. The books recommend the same type of bland diet, lots of starches, milk, protein and a coating like Pepto Bismal.

After two months of bland foods, I asked again if this diet was deficient in nutrients. The doctor said it would just take time to get better and that I would be fine. I tried to put vegetables back in my diet, but it caused my stomach so much pain that I had to again stop eating vegetables and fruits.

Then, I suddenly became sensitive to certain laundry detergents. The natural detergents in the health food store gave me no problems, but it was impossible to walk down an ordinary grocery stores' detergent aisle because of the irritation caused by the odors and fragrances.

My clothes, which were made of synthetic materials, suffocated my skin causing me to feel itchy. The sheets on my bed were 60% polyester and 40% cotton and irritated my skin. I switched all of my clothes and sheets to 100% cotton and immediately felt relief.

I could not walk into our porch with its brand new mauve carpet; the sickening synthetic carpet vapors lay heavy in the air. The black-inked newspapers and books gave off metallic odors making it impossible to read. My mother-in-law told me she too had become sensitive to chemicals when she was exposed to a high level of ammonia while working. She was bedridden for months, yet she made it through that hard time and was able to get on with her life.

My mother and mother-in-law took turns living with us to care for my daughter and me.

Fourteen weeks later I became too ill to walk. I was resigned to lying on the floor. My jaw hurt so badly I was unable to read Jacky her bedtime story. Sitting up now was too painful for my stomach. I had to buy pants two sizes too big to prevent pressure on my stomach. My face was covered with tears all day long. My bedroom walls set a barrier from the outside with closed doors as warnings to go away. I did not want my husband or daughter seeing me in this shattered way—a bag of tortured worn-out bones. I wanted it all to end—to just step out of this living hell. I asked God over and over—why me? I screamed angrily with hands flying in the air, "Please God, help me!"

My mother was having a nervous breakdown seeing me this way. My husband wanted to put me in the hospital. I would not go because from my experiences over the last seven years the doctors were not helpful.

The pain was so unbearable that I used mental images to escape. I closed my eyes and imagined hearing the sounds of the ocean waves crashing into each speck of white sand. The deep blue ocean turned to turquoise then green with bright white foam bubbling on top. I felt the warm soft sand surrounding my toes. A clear blue sky with a powerful sun, far too radiant to look into, beat on my body. I sat down. Life was wonderful here. I didn't want to go back. Sea gulls flew overhead gliding on the cool breeze. Pigeons strutted, their bodies cast off rainbows as they twisted their fine necks. Most people think pigeons are disgusting dirty birds and compare them to rats. I don't agree. Why can't people look a little closer at the pigeon's iridescent neck and see it shimmering in the sun's rays—changing colors from purple, to blue, green and yellow?

Seconds later I was back to the cruel reality of life. I was trying hard to look closer at my options through yellow-tinged eyes with pale yellow dried skin. I was a sickly 98 pound body with hair falling out. What was the easiest way to end life? Pictures of high bridges, loaded guns and graves flashed through my mind.

I called my father and insisted that he go to the library and health food stores to do research. I told him I was dying and I didn't know why. "You have to help me Dad, no one else is." He said, "I don't know how to help you or where to start. I'm not a doctor. I don't know what to do."

It was now twenty weeks and I was only getting worse. I knew I would die if I did not get help. I had to look closer at my options because no one knew how to help me.

We traveled to San Diego, California, praying that San Diego would have more open-minded and better types of therapy. Just to sit up during the six hour plane trip was torture, but once I arrived I felt better because of the sunshine and ocean air. With high spirits I immediately went through the phone book's yellow pages looking for health food stores so I could ask for information on where to get help.

A few of the recommended doctors had pieces of the health puzzle but none had a complete solution. Some wanted me to take saunas, vitamins (including Vitamin C intravenous therapy), acupuncture, juices, sprouts, reflexology, while others wanted to test my blood for toxicity. None of these ideas seemed complete and I knew there was something missing.

At this same time, I was now becoming allergic to chicken, turkey, and white rice (the only foods I was still able to eat). I searched for new foods, believing I was allergic to the usual ones. This was how I came upon a meat market that specialized in different types of animals: buffalo and pheasant to just name a few. I told the butcher the problems I was having and why I came to his store. The nice man behind the meat counter said he knew of a customer, a woman whose son had allergies like mine. I said I would like to talk to her to get some ideas on how to deal with the allergies. He would get her telephone number for me if I would like. I said yes and (thank goodness) he got the number for me.

THE NATURAL HEALTH PHILOSOPHY

One week later I called her. Her story was encouraging. She told me she had found some concentrated whole food products that appeared to both alleviate her son's allergies and strengthen her eight-year-old son's body. She said, "He is tolerating the environment and foods much better." She invited me to one of the food company's product meetings. I was too sick to go alone so my parents took me, but only after I cried and begged my disbelieving father to come.

Unexpectedly, the first thing we noticed at the meeting was that all the people attending looked healthy. I was angry and decided that this can't be. I thought the meeting was for sick people. As I lay in pain on the floor in the back of the meeting room, I heard a strong woman speaker talk about how she had been very ill until she found these whole food products and the natural philosophy of health. She explained a completely different health approach than I had ever heard.

WHAT DID SHE SAY?

Principle #1: The body can heal itself if it is provided with the right nutrition. (The body has different nutritional needs for each part of the body and all these parts need to be properly nourished.)

Principle #2: The body is designed to obtain its nutrition from whole foods—not from isolated vitamins, amino acids, and chemicals, but from the entire food. (When our creator made our bodies, he provided us whole foods to use for repairing, building, and creating energy.)

Principle #3: You and you alone have to take responsibility for your own health. No one else is going to do it for you. (Listen to your body and it will tell you what to do. Study, ponder and then apply what you learn. Your body is the best monitor as to the value of any program or system. If you need to improve your nutrition, then learn about foods and whole food concentrates.)

These ideas were logical but scary. Think of all the food substitutes people take, like vitamins. My father made me swallow vitamins from the age of seven to make sure I had all the nutrients. Could this have set me up for my ensuing problems?

One day a friend of ours, a young doctor just out of medical school, stayed overnight at our house. As he was eating breakfast cereal with us the next morning, he happened to read the label of the enriched product and said "I learned in lab class that our bodies do not know the difference between isolated vitamins and whole foods. Once you swallow this enriched cereal your body has been tricked and you benefit from all the added nutrients."

The doctor's statement was interesting. It was the opposite of what the woman at the natural health meeting had said. She said you cannot trick your body as it is extremely intelligent and knows the difference between whole foods and chemicals. The nutrients in food need to hold hands and build with each other for us to benefit from them all.

4

CHINESE

For 5000 years the Chinese have used herbs and plants for healing the body. They are known for experimenting with plants, herbs, fruits and nuts in order to better understand their relationship with our nutritional needs. They have studied and recorded the effects on the body of as many as 10,000 plants. What evolved from this meticulous study was a philosophy of regeneration; the knowledge that the body could bring itself to a "perfect state" by using exact whole food plant combinations that nourish the entire body.

To the ancient Chinese hunger and disease were very much the same—left untended both resulted in poor health and imbalance. Illness meant our body hungered for nourishment. When nourishment is provided by whole food herbs, vegetables, and fruit, our body will use them to function properly, regain health, and prevent disease. This observation was fascinating and I read everything I could get my hands on to understand this different concept on how the human body functions. They believed in a Yin-Yang (negative and positive balance) system. You easily can understand this system of opposite relationships in life; because it is so obvious, you see it everywhere once it is described.

"The Chinese system of Yin and Yang, the East Indian Ayurveda system, are examples of naturalistic systems—all of them known in the jargon as `hot-cold systems' in which the disequilibrium can be corrected by restoring the balance of elements in the individual's life or body. In this group, the responsibility for becoming ill usually rests with the patient"[1]

[1] Dr. Cecil Helman, "What is Medical Anthropology?" *Mims Magazine* [London] 1 April-15 August 1980.

I understood that life is full of Yin and Yang. Intuitively I knew this was an absolute truth; therefore, food must also have Yin and Yang properties to balance our bodies.

YIN	YANG
Cold	Hot
Inhale	Exhale
Regressive	Aggressive
Passive	Domineering
Bland	Spicy
Sour	Sweet
Female	Male

Additionally, the Chinese believe in a flow of nature that is divided into five parts or elements: fire, earth, metal, water, and wood. The illustration shows how the five elements relate to five systems of our body.

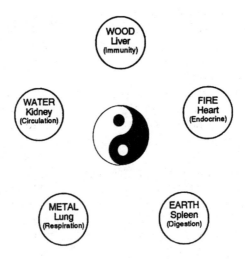

The Chinese consider that all five elements have to be balanced (yin-yang) with each other and within animals, nature, plants, and humans. The optimum balance results in a harmonious healthy condition. I liked the idea that our bodies could be strengthened by eating particular foods for the different systems in our body such as digestive, respiratory, immune, endocrine and circulatory. For example, digestion could be strengthened by eating cinnamon.

Upon studying the nutrients of herbs versus common vegetables (carrots, celery, broccoli, etc.), I discovered that herbs have a higher concentration of vitamins and minerals. I also found that the idea of eating specific foods to strengthen specific systems wasn't alien to our western world. For instance, the American Cancer Society now is finding that broccoli and spinach strengthen the esophagus against cancer, whereas cauliflower and cabbage strengthen the respiratory system. These findings are very similar to conclusions of a Chinese study on more than two thousand plants done 5,000 years ago.

DEAN BLACK

Can someone die from eating food? Dean Black nearly did. Because he had food allergies, his body went into anaphylactic shock after he ate some strawberries. Fortunately, just before his body shut down he was able to drive to a hospital where his doctor diagnosed the problem and immediately counteracted the shock by injecting adrenaline into Dean's body.

Spurred by this near death experience, Dean went to a Chinese herbal doctor in 1979 to seek an understanding of his problem. The herbal doctor told him not to worry about the allergies being a permanent condition and that the way to alleviate the allergy problem was to eat some whole food herbs. He followed the herbal doctor's suggestions and within two weeks found that he not only got rid of the food allergies, but his hay fever had also disappeared. His health improvement was so positive that Dean decided to study the difference in health philosophy between Chinese traditional healers and western medical doctors. He concluded that:

"For centuries now, two different kinds of healers have contended for the health-care market. Today we might call them natural healers and medical doctors. In general, natural healers seek to sustain the body's natural processes, while medical doctors seek to replace them with drugs or machines.

"By looking at the body as a whole, a Chinese Doctor would take into account, for example, the patient's

1. Complexion
2. Likes-dislikes
3. Smell
4. Tastes
5. Appearance
6. Gait

"The doctor could then determine the patient's balance, expressed as the relationship between two opposites—yin (calmness) and yang (activity). He would decide if the patient were too yin (tired all the time, walks with shoulders hunched over, sleeps long hours) or too yang (hyperactive, can't sleep, has destructive relationships). Then the Chinese Doctor would simply adjust various aspects of the patient's diet and behavior in order to re-balance him. *This balancing is the key to healing.*"

How does an individual create this balance? Through knowledge. Dean says, "We must look at disease or other problems as a challenge that will teach us the wisdom we need to create balance and good health. If we view challenge as our teacher, it will teach us wisdom. This partnership between challenge and wisdom will create a series of steps leading to well being."

Dean also explains how classical scientists follow a theory of taking things apart. The human body is taken apart and studied, cell by cell, until in comparison, the organism becomes infinite and contains an infinity of cells. This infinity of cells becomes Chaos in current scientific context.

By putting the body in its whole working context with whole foods, five senses, the mind and spirit we can then help heal ourselves. Let's look at the substances we put in our bodies.

They can be broken down into four categories:

1. Whole fruits and vegetables which are regenerative and help to maintain and support health
2. Vitamins which are isolated chemicals.
3. Medicinal Herbs which have a limited use such as 3 months or less.
4. Pharmaceutical Drugs which substitute for the body functions.

AN EXAMPLE OF SUBSTITUTION AND REGENERATION

Take the example of our digestive system. For it to operate properly our digestion system needs hydrochloric acid. If you have digestion problems, you go to the doctor for an examination. After examining you, the doctor finds your digestive problems are due to an insufficient amount of hydrochloric acid. He then prescribes hydrochloric acid pills for you to take. You buy the pills and take them. It works! Your stomach problems seem to be gone—that is until the hydrochloric acid in the stomach is used up, then the ache returns and back you go to the doctor for more pills.

You know the body is a self-regulating mechanism and is designed to create its own hydrochloric acid when given the proper nutrition. So the question is: Does this *substitution for a body function* solve the problem of the body's inability to produce hydrochloric acid? No, it is a *substitution for the acid* so the body does not have to create it on its own. Unfortunately, *substitution tends to create some negative effects*. First, it appears to create a greater weakness of the body function. If a body function isn't used, it weakens until it dies, like your muscles. Second, when the function ceases to operate, the body appears to create a *dependency on the substitute*. Third, substitutes rarely only affect the function they are intended to help. There are almost always side effects, many of which may be dangerous to good health. If you take a substitute to help with high blood pressure, it may also cause nausea. You take a substitute for nausea, and that may cause dizziness. You take a substitute for dizziness and it may cause who knows what. It goes on and on.

Now lets apply the Chinese philosophy of *regeneration* to this same example of digestion. The Chinese found from experience that certain food herbs feed specific systems of the body. From this information, they developed "food" formulas to feed specific systems of the body. What foods do you use? My study suggests that you try the whole food herb formulas the Chinese have used for years to feed the digestive system. You eat these food herbs. Your body then takes the nutrients from those herb foods and feeds the digestive system. The digestive system utilizes those nutrients and is once again able to produce hydrochloric acid. This is *regeneration*!

Yes, I could understand this simple solution to health—*regeneration though wholes*. The key was the word *whole*. We have been in a dark sunless laboratory too long, looking too closely at molecules and chemicals, taking apart, isolating, and trying to understand the pieces. When it is actually the *whole* system that counts.

As I continued listening with fascination, I began to believe that what the speaker was saying was true. After the lecture was over, I asked the speaker "Where do I start? I'm in so much pain. Are the foods going to make my stomach hurt more?" She said, "Yes, it's going to hurt as your body regenerates." This was amazing. The pain I'd been hiding from was really a good omen. Pain was my bodies' way of telling me something was wrong. I had to look at pain not as a negative but as a positive sign. This was a completely different way to think about my body; therefore, I had to revise my thinking about ways to get better.

The first thing I did was to ask my mother to go to as many meetings as she could on the whole foods and to get phone numbers of women who had suffered similar problems as mine. She did and I was able to call from Ohio to Seattle to San Francisco to San Diego to talk to them and discuss how they ate and what whole food herbs they used to improve their health. They recommended books, diets and herbs. I needed this support from others who had gone through the same suffering I did and had gotten their health back. Also the women using the foods were honest and open in teaching me about the concept of detoxification and regeneration though diet.

I found the following wonderful paper written by Ede Koenig about detoxification and regeneration through diet and read it over and over. I've included it for your benefit.

5

DETOXIFICATION AND REGENERATION THROUGH DIET

By Ede Koenig

A great deal of confusion in the field of nutrition is caused by the failure to properly understand and interpret the symptoms and the changes which follow the implementation of a natural diet.

The highest quality of food is found in natural, whole and raw foods. All the enzymes are found intact. The amino acids are in their finest form. The minerals, vitamins, carbohydrates, trace elements and "life force" are present. The "life force," in turn, is capable of reproducing healthy tissue. When the quality of food coming into the body is of higher quality than the tissues which the body is made of, the body begins to discard the lower grade materials and tissues to make room for the superior materials which it uses to make new and healthier tissue.

This is the plan of Nature. The body is very selective and always will be unless our interference is too great. Only then do we fail to recover and degenerate further into disease. The self-curing nature of many conditions such as colds, fevers, cuts, swellings, injuries, pain, etc., furnishes endless examples of how the body tends toward health—always—unless we do something to stop the process.

What are the symptoms or signs which become evident when we first begin to omit the lower grade foods and instead introduce superior foods—those which are more alive, more natural than we are accustomed to? When the use of the toxic stimulant such as coffee, tea, chocolate, or cocoa is suddenly stopped, headaches are common and a letdown occurs. This is

due to the discard by the body of the toxins called caffeine
and theobromide which are removed from body tissues and
transported through the blood stream during its many bodily
rounds. Before the noxious agents reach their final destination
for elimination, these irritants register in our consciousness as
pain—in other words, headache.

The letdown is due to the slower action of the heart—the
resting phase which follows the more rapid heart action forced
upon the body by certain poisons called stimulants (that can
be in the form of drug medications). The more rapid
heartbeat (or pulse) produces a feeling of exhilaration, and the
slower action produces a depressed state of mind. Usually
within three days the symptoms vanish and we feel stronger
due to the recuperation which follows.

To a lesser extent, the same process occurs when we
abandon lower quality foods and replace them with better
foods. Lower quality foods have undergone more preparation;
spices, salt and other ingredients have been added, which then
tend to be more stimulating than less prepared and more
natural foods.

Animal foods and products, such as meat, fowl, fish,
cheese, milk, eggs, etc., are more stimulating than seeds, nuts,
grains, and vegetable proteins. Consequently, the withdrawal
of stimulation which follows the abandonment of animal
foods produces a slower heart action—a resting phase—which
registers in the mind as relaxation or a decrease in energy.
This initial letdown lasts about ten days or slightly longer and
is followed by an increase of strength, a feeling of diminishing
stress, and greater well-being.

Now, let us return to the symptoms which occur in the
process of regeneration. The person who starts a better diet,
stays on it for three days to a week and then quits, will say,
"Oh! I felt better on the old diet—the new one made me feel
weak." He failed because he didn't give his body a chance to
adjust and complete its first phase of action—recuperation. If
he had waited awhile longer, he would have begun to feel
better than before he started.

During this initial phase (lasting about ten days on the
average to several weeks in others), the vital energies which are
usually in the periphery or external part of the body, such as
the muscles and skin, begin to move to the vital internal
organs and start reconstruction.

This shunting of much of the power to the internal organs produces a feeling of less energy in the muscles, which the mind interprets as some weakness. Actually, the power is increased, but most of it is being used for rebuilding the more important organs and less of it is available for muscular work. Any weakness which is felt here is not true weakness, but merely is a deployment of forces to the more important internal parts. Here it is important for the person to stop wasting energy, and to rest and sleep more. This is a crucial phase, and if the person resorts to stimulants of any kind, he will abort and defeat the regenerative intent of the body.

It is important that he have patience and faith and just wait it out, and after awhile he will get increasing strength which will exceed by far what he felt before he began the new program. Success in recovery or improvement of health hinges upon the correct understanding of this point—realizing that the body is using its main energies in more important internal work and not wasting it in external work involving muscle movements.

Be wise—take it easy here and relax. Just coast in your work and social obligations until you're out of the woods. As one continues on the improved diet and gradually raises the food quality, interesting symptoms begin to occur. The body begins a process called "retracting". The cellular intelligence reasons something like this:

"Oh! Look at all this fine material coming in. How wonderful! Now we have a chance to get rid of this old garbage and build a beautiful new house. Let's get started immediately.

"Let's get this excess bile out of the liver and gallbladder and send it to the intestines for elimination. Let's get this sludge moving out of the arteries, veins and capillaries. These smelly, gassy, brain-stupefying masses have been here too long—out with them! These arthritic deposits in the joints need cleaning up. Let's get these irritating food preservatives, sleeping pills, aspirins, and drugs out of the way, along with these other masses of fat which have made life so burdensome for us for so long.

During the first phase, called catabolism, the accent is on elimination, or breaking down of tissue. The body begins to clean house—in short, to remove the garbage deposited in all the tissues—everywhere.

During this period, the body "removes the ashes from the furnace preparatory to getting a better fire." Here, the accentuation is on the removal of the gross and immediate body obstructions. Wastes are discarded more rapidly, then new tissue is made from the new food. This becomes evident as weight loss. This persists for awhile and is then followed by the second phase—stabilization.

Here the weight remains more or less stable. During this phase the amount of waste material being discarded daily is equal to the amount of tissue which is being formed and replaced by the newer, more vital food. This occurs after the excess of obstructing material in the tissues has been removed.

This stage persists for awhile and is then followed by a third phase—a build-up period, called anabolism, wherein weight starts to go up, even though the diet is lower in calories than it was before.

At this point, much or more of the interfering wastes have already been discarded—the tissue which has formed since the diet is raised in quality, is more durable and does not break down easily. Also, new tissues are now being formed faster.

This is due to the improved assimilation made possible by the ceasing of wrong food-combining. The body's need for the usual amounts of food decreases, and we are able to maintain our weight and increased energies with less food. Many are able to function very efficiently on two meals a day and eventually even on one meal a day.

As the body progressively increases in efficiency and decreases in tissue breakdown in the body, so do we gradually need less and less food to maintain life. The higher the percentage of whole and raw foods one lives on, the slower the rate of tissue deterioration. A sick body requires a gradual, carefully worked-out entry into this stage, where one is able to live on a 100 percent uncooked raw diet.

Returning to the symptoms which occur on a superior nutritional program, people who have had tendencies in the past toward recurring skin rashes or eruptions will frequently tend to eliminate poisons and harmful drugs through the skin with new rashes or eruptions. If they go to a doctor, now, who is unfamiliar with this aspect of nutrition, he will diagnose it as an allergy. They ask, "How come I'm eating better now than I ever did before, and instead I'm getting worse?"

They don't understand that the body is "retracting." The skin is getting more alive and active. It's throwing out more poisons more rapidly now that the body is building more power which is saved from those hard-to-digest meals which have been discontinued. These toxins being discarded are saving you from more serious disease, which will result if you keep them in your body too much longer—possibly hepatitis, kidney disorder, blood disease, heart disease, arthritis, nerve degenerations, or even cancer—depending on your heredity or structural weaknesses. Be happy you're paying your bills now in an easy-payment plan.

With some, colds which haven't appeared for a long time may occur, or even fevers; this is nature's way of housecleaning.

Understand that these actions are constructive, even though unpleasant at the moment. Don't try to stop these symptoms by the use of certain drugs, or even massive doses of vitamins which will act as drugs in huge concentrations. These symptoms are part of a curing process—don't try to cure a cure.

Don't expect to go on an ascending scale of quality—that improving your diet will make you feel better and better each day until you reach perfection. The body is cyclical in nature (in a circadian rhythm), and health returns in a series of gradually diminishing cycles. For example, you start a better diet and for awhile you feel much better. After some time, a symptom occurs—you may feel nauseous for a day and have diarrhea with a foul-smelling stool. After a day, you feel even better and all goes fine for awhile. Then you suddenly develop a cold, feel chills, and lose your appetite. After about two or three days (assuming you don't take drugs or do anything else about it), you suddenly recover and feel better than you did for years.

Let us say this well-being continues for two months, when you suddenly develop an itch or rash. You still don't take anything for it. This rash flares up, gets worse and continues for ten days, and suddenly subsides. Immediately after this you find that your hepatitis is gone and your energy has increased more than ever before.

The rash became an outlet for the poisons in the liver which produced the hepatitis. This is how recovery occurs—

like the cycles in the Dow-Jones Average at the beginning of a bull market.

You feel better, a reaction occurs and you don't feel as well for a short time. You recover and go higher for awhile. Then another reaction occurs, milder than the last. You recover and go even higher. And so it goes.

Each reaction milder than the first as the body becomes purer, each becoming shorter in duration and being followed by a longer and longer period of feeling better than ever before, until you reach a level plateau of radiant health.

The first laws we must learn to obey are the laws of Nature. We must learn to eat simple, pure and natural food, properly prepared and combined, and our bodies in return will cast off all the evil we have taken in during our lives. Nowhere is the principle of forgiveness of sins more manifest than here—in our own bodies—when we forsake our evil and destructive ways of eating (the defiling of the temple of the soul). God (or Nature, if you prefer) gives us a whole new chance for a new glorious life. All repentance must begin here in the body—through the purer diet and natural foods. Then, just have faith, sit back, and watch what happens.

* * * * *

Understanding the above, I knew I had to completely trust my body to go through the cleansing process, this miracle of transforming every cell, muscle and tissue of my body, to make way for better health though diet. (By Ede Koenig)

My first cleanse cycle produced lots of diarrhea, coughing up of phlegm, swollen lymph nodes in my throat and under my arms, peeling and yellow colored nails, lots of hair fell out, canker sores, running nose, miserably cold hands and feet, weakness in the arms and legs and a need to sleep long hours. All of this overwhelmed me so much that I would get on my telephone and call other people to reconfirm that what I was going through was truly a healing crisis. The others had suffered similar cleanse cycles indicating I was no different than anyone else and I would just have to hang in there and go at my own pace toward health.

My pace toward transforming my body was similar to a turtle's pace. I hate pain so much I reduced my intake of healthy food when I could no longer tolerate the cleansing. But afterwards started back up when I felt better. I knew even though I had many systems to cleanse I was becoming better because parts of my body were stronger. I was able to stand on my feet longer. The burning on top of my skin was disappearing. My jaw pain, temporomandibular joint dysfunction (TMJD), was slowly going away. At the precise moment I was able to walk from the parking lot to the health food store all by myself I knew that I would succeed. Although I would have to go though much hard work, pain and discipline to get better.

One thing I discovered was that charting my health was an excellent way to find when my good days (or bad days) would occur. Interestingly, as my health improved, the chart appeared to form a spiral.

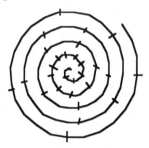

I believe that when a person is sick their body feels rotten everyday. Look at the diagram. The center of the spiral (fewest good days) shows the starting point of a healing crisis. The healing crisis initiates the start of a cleansing and rebuilding period and appears as many bad days followed by some good days. This chart shows how the bad days continue to decrease as one grows healthier, i.e., moves away from the center of the spiral. When you reach the outer edge you should not feel these cycles anymore. For instance, I would feel rotten six days a week and good one day. This lasted for a month repeating on every Thursday as the cycles were extremely predictable as long as I was eating a better diet. The following month I felt good two days a week. As time passed I ultimately reached a good state of health for the entire seven days of the week. This took about one year.

HERING'S THREE LAWS

That the body heals from head to toe and from inside to outside are the laws of the homeopathic physician Constantine Hering who lived from 1800-1880.

1. **First Law:** Symptoms of a chronic disease disappear in a definite order when the patient is properly treated. Symptoms usually disappear in the reverse order of their appearance—the most recent symptom disappears first; then an earlier symptom manifests only to abate when the proper remedy is given. This process continues until all the unresolved disease conditions are eliminated, even though some may go back to early childhood. This is called the progression of symptoms.

2. **Second Law:** Symptoms tend to move from the interior of the body toward the periphery, or skin. This law functions because of the body's attempt to preserve itself. If a disease that produces morbid matter can't be eliminated, the body tries to deposit the residues of this condition in as harmless an area as possible. The skin is one of the safest, but the various connective tissues and joints are also frequently used by the body for this purpose. Only when the disease process is overpowering does the body allow it to invade vital organs, and even then the body makes every possible attempt to keep the disease processes out of the heart and brain.

3. **Third Law:** Symptoms move from the top of the body downward, disappearing first from the head, then from the thigh, then to the knee, ankle and foot. We frequently encounter this last pattern, wherein the pain will go from the abdomen into the hip, then thigh, then knee, and then in and out the foot.

My own healing followed this precise order. First my mind started functioning smoother. I had clearer thoughts and memory improvement. While this was happening, my arms and legs remained extremely weak.

During a lecture on homeopathy, I heard the lecturer mention Herring's law. He said "My daughter had chicken pox and she healed in this order: internal mouth sores went away first, followed by sores going away from head down to toes."

6

PROTEIN

A woman I called in Los Angeles told me confidently that if I eliminated all animal foods (chicken, fish, eggs, dairy, etc.) from my diet I would become healthy quicker. She had seen many people become healthier when they quit eating animal products. I was shocked at this comment believing at that time animal protein was one of our major food groups! I called all over the United States to get other opinions, even going to the book store to see if nutritional books agreed with eliminating animal products from our diets. Out of the 67 health books I examined, the majority were for taking out animal protein completely or at least cutting back on the amount eaten. I found that some people were following a low animal protein diet even though they did not understand why animal protein may not be that good. I asked my Doctor what he thought about a zero animal protein diet. He said, "If you take out your animal protein, what will you eat? You will go hungry! There's not enough foods out there. Taking animal protein out is a terrible idea."

On the other hand, my nutritional advisor thought it was a great idea. He said it was a myth that our bodies need so much protein. We can get all we need from fruits, vegetables, nuts and seeds. He said, "Our bodies needed roughly 12 grams a day."

How did our country arrive at our daily needs of protein? A committee called the National Academy of Sciences, Food and Nutrition Board recommended our Dietary Allowances.

"Its interesting to learn how the committee arrives at these recommended allowances," said Frances Moore Lappé in the book *Diet for a Small Planet*. I agree with her. The way they went about our protein requirements' test is dumbfounding!

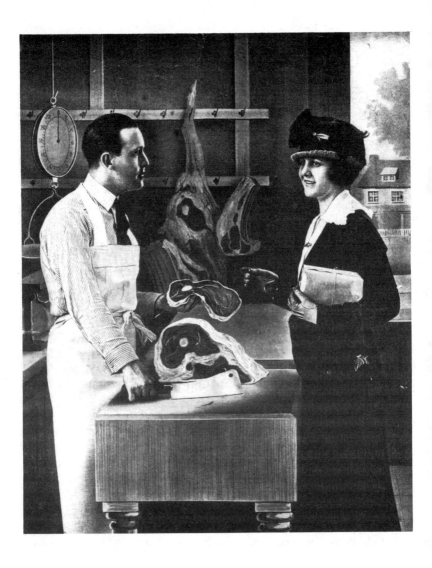

Incredibly, the committee calculated our daily protein needs solely by using scientific data obtained in lab tests which examined urine and feces for protein content. Why not base protein needs on the protein content of the ideal food?

Why didn't they look at the start of human life, the natural source of food, human mothers' milk? Or what about looking at death, or health? See which tribe or people live healthier, longer lives? Examine their protein intake.

To come up with the recommended allowance for an entire population, the committee followed four steps:

Step 1. Estimate average need. Since nitrogen is a characteristic and relatively constant component of protein, scientists can measure protein by measuring nitrogen. To determine how much protein humans need, experimenters put subjects on a protein-free diet. They then measured how much nitrogen was lost in urine and feces.

Step 2. Adjust for individual differences.

Step 3. Adjust for normal eating.

Step 4. Adjust for protein usability. Therefore, the allowance of 42 grams of protein for a 154-pound man is pushed up to 56 grams because it is assumed that only 75 percent of what is eaten is actually used. For a 128-pound woman, the average American female, the corresponding allowance is 44 grams.[1]

The test for protein is based on the amount of nitrogen lost. Positive nitrogen balance is completely maintained in a vegetable based diet.

Nathan Pritikin, his book *The Pritikin Program*, found that you don't have to eat animals and could get adequate protein from a plant-based diet. He tells us, "One of the longest studies testing low protein intake in humans was done by Walter Kempner, MD, of Duke University. In 1949, he presented the findings of his rice-fruit diet at the American College of Physicians 30th annual session. Kempner's diet had 2000 calories, consisting of 4 percent protein, all from plant sources, 2.3 percent fat, and 93 percent carbohydrates, both complex and simple, and no cholesterol. Only 20 grams of protein were provided, which was adequate to maintain adults in positive nitrogen balance.

"Seven hundred seventy-seven Highlanders in Papua, New Guinea, have been studied extensively because of their very-low protein diet (4.4%) which by western standards would seem to guarantee malnutrition, ill health, and protein deficiency. The New Guineans have none of these conditions,

---

[1] Frances Moore Lappe, *Diet for a Small Planet,* p.170.

and are not only healthy, muscular, and do heavy work, but are free of heart disease, diabetes, hypertension, and breast and colon cancer.For generations their diet has been limited to sweet potatoes and sweet-potato leaves with a pig feast every 2 or 3 years.

"The amino acid intake pattern, as compared with the FDA recommended pattern, appears to be grossly inadequate and nitrogen-balance studies by Dr. Oomen found New Guineans of all ages to be in a negative nitrogen balance."

Is it possible that there could be something wrong with our conclusions from the positive nitrogen balance test? Look at it this way. Our protein requirements were determined in the laboratory, not by studying healthy animals physiologically similar to us. The ape and the monkey have a raw diet of nuts, seeds, fruits and vegetables that contain about 12 grams of protein a day. Instead, they have us eating a diet for a vulture. How many people are going to suffer before scientists revise their thinking and re-evaluate the nitrogen test? The following would be a normal animal diet for a so-called healthy America.

Meal	**Food**	**Protein Content** (grams approx.)
Breakfast:		
	Cereal	3
	Low Fat Milk	8
		11
Lunch:		
	Tuna Sandwich, 3 oz.	
	Bread	2
	Tuna	25
	Lettuce	1
	Tomato	0.5
	Milk	8
		36.5
Dinner:		
	Chicken, 3 oz.	23
	Broccoli, 1 cup, cooked	5
	Corn on the Cob, cooked	3
	Coke	0
		31
Total protein for the day		78.6

Americans eat on the average 80 grams of protein a day. They exceed the recommended 30 grams because every time they think of a meal, they base it on the supposed need to eat animals or their by-products, such as hot dogs, hamburgers, pork chops, eggs, cheese, milk, etc. We have been bombarded on TV and in other advertisements by the Meat Industry and the Dairy Council telling us that animal by-products are good for us.

I went to the library in Broomall, Pennsylvania, to research diet. There was a file there on nutrition. Fifty percent (50%) of this file was filled with nutritional advice from the Meat Industry and the Dairy Council.

The following is a normal vegetarian diet with protein content.

Meal	Food	Protein Content (grams approx.)
Breakfast:		
	Bananas (2)	2.2
Lunch:		
	Avocado Sandwich	
	Rice Bread	7.5
	Avocado	2.2
	Tomato	0.5
	Lettuce	0.4
		10.6
Dinner:		
	Broccoli	5
	Corn	3
	Salad	0.2
	Carrot	1.1
		9.3
Total for the Day		22.1

I have found from my research that the fewer animal by-products you eat, the less chance you have of getting a disease. So, how should you get your protein? Let's take a look at a human mothers' milk—in one cup, there are 2.56 grams of protein. Many nutritionists forget that the 6 percent of total calories in protein present in breast milk is adequate for the fast growth of human babies who double their birth weight in the first six months of life. During no other period in life is there as great a protein requirement. An average baby drinks three cups a day, which is a total of 7.68 grams of protein. When he gets all his teeth, by the age of 15 months, he will be put on a diet completely different in nutritional content from his mothers' milk. He will be eating table food, and his protein intake will become 25 grams, or more, a day, which is suggested by the National Academy of Science. This triples his protein consumption.

If our children were kept on a diet free of animal products, they would achieve the protein closest to human mothers' milk as well as meet the government's protein requirements.

But when animal products are added, the child's protein intake goes up by 64 grams, many times higher than human mothers' milk.

Another misconception regarding protein is that you must receive all the essential amino acids at one meal for our bodies to absorb the protein. If you wish to receive your protein from a plant-based diet then make sure that you eat 22 amino acids (Tryptophan, Isoleucine, Lysine, Valine, Threonine, Sulfur, etc.) at one meal in correct amounts. Also, we are told that our only food source of complete protein is animals—unless you use a vegetarian diet that utilizes complementary foods like beans and rice to receive amino acids.

Frances Moore Lappé (a food expert who began her studies in 1969) writes in the second edition of her book, *Diet For A Small Planet*, that "with a healthy varied diet, concern about eating a complete protein at each meal is not necessary for most of us. The body stores amino acids within its own pool for weeks. The body calls upon the missing amino acids when it goes to form a complete protein." Thus she dispels the myth that complementing protein is necessary for most people on a low or meatless diet.

It is very important to eat a healthy varied diet of different colors of fruit, vegetables, nuts, and seeds to make sure you receive the building blocks, but not necessarily at one meal. Also remember that enzymes are the activators of the protein chain so you must eat an enzyme rich diet.

Now that we have cleared up the laboratory myths, lets look at practical knowledge. You have heard the expression "three strikes and you're out." What about fourteen strikes (or reasons) we stop eating animal products.

1. PROTEIN IN ANIMALS IS TOO CONCENTRATED FOR HUMAN NEEDS.

Dr. Dean Black says, "Our diets are too high in protein." It is my opinion that the protein content of human mothers' milk is a good gauge of our protein requirements—it is only 6% protein and at a time when the rate of human (baby) growth is maximum.

Food must be balanced—not too much isolated sugar or pure protein. Foods must have a combination of protein and sugar, like vegetables and fruit. Staying between the two extremes creates balance.

Sugar Fruit	Vegetables Isolated
Candy	protein
	Animals

2. THERE IS NO FIBER IN ANIMAL PRODUCTS.

"Fiber acts like a broom in your intestines sweeping things along. Without it, waste gets blocked up, and the length of time your food takes to pass though your colon is greatly increased"[1]

This is particularly true if your diet contains animal fat. Animal fats are solid at body temperature and may clog up your intestines as grease clogs up a drain. Animal protein and its wrong kinds of fat go hand in hand. No matter how hard you try to cut off fat you can't eliminate it, because the fat is dispersed throughout the meat.

Animal protein takes two to three days to pass through the colon. Vegetables and fruit take twenty-four hours. Could these extra two days of residence time for the animal foods allow toxic wastes to develop in the colon? Try this. Put some

---

[1] Adelle Davis, *Let's Get Well,* p. 153.

chicken in a container and leave it on your counter top for two days at room temperature. Room temperature is about 20 to 30 degrees cooler than our body's inside temperature; therefore, the chicken will be in a more "friendly environment" than in our bodies. Would you still eat that chicken? Of course not. Probably, you wouldn't even risk smelling it. But isn't this what we do unintentionally with our "standard American stopped up plumbing" bodies? Now let's leave a piece of fruit, say an apple or banana, out for one day or more. Eating this fruit is no problem. We do it all the time and don't even think about it.

The nutritionists tell everyone "Dietary fiber appears to aid in reducing colon and rectal cancer!" We need to realize animal products have no fiber in them.

3. MEAT FREQUENTLY CONTAINS DANGEROUS CHEMICALS.

Animals may be kept alive and fattened by the use of tranquilizers, hormones and antibiotics. One of the hormones used in past years, a hormone known as Diethylstilbestrol (Des), has been shown to be carcinogenic and has been banned in 32 countries, yet to my knowledge, it continues to be used by the US meat industry today. This is because the FDA estimates it saves meat producers more than $500 million annually.

I was extremely surprised when I discovered that fruits and vegetables were lower in pesticide residue than animal products.

4. RESEARCH HAS SHOWN THAT A HIGH PROTEIN DIET BASED UPON MEAT CAN CAUSE URINARY CALCIUM LOSS.

Dr. Airola reports that high protein intake disrupts the calcium-phosphate ratio since meat has 22 times more phosphorous then calcium. This leads to osteoporosis.

5. EXCESS PROTEIN CAN LEAD TO PREMATURE AGING.

Hormones in animals bring on old age quicker and speed up childhood development. Children on a meat diet grow larger earlier because of the hormones in animals. The more protein in the diet the sooner a feminine child will start her menstruation.

Animal protein, with its high fat content, is related to disease, especially heart disease. "As early as 1961, the *Journal of the American Medical Association* stated that 90 to 97% of heart disease (which accounts for approximately half of the deaths in this country) could be prevented by a vegetarian diet."[1] "The relationship between a high animal flesh and fat diet and colon cancer is becoming quite evident. Remember, the only place you receive the wrong kind of fat (cholesterol) is from animals. Fruits, vegetables, grains, nuts, and seeds have only the right kind of fats (no cholesterol) for the human body."

6. WE ARE EATING DISEASED AND MALNOURISHED ANIMALS.

"A 1972 USDA report lists carcasses that have passed inspection after the diseased parts were removed. Some examples included almost 100,000 cows with eye cancer and 3,596,302 cases with abscessed liver. To surgically remove the cancer site is missing the point. In a condition of malignant cancer, the illness is not simply in the local tumor, for in the case of malignant carcinoma a frequent prerequisite is an organism which is systematically ill. Therefore, when you consume meat, you cannot be certain that the animal would not have died from some disease, had it not been slaughtered to end up on your dinner table!"[2]

Feeding the animals dead enzymeless food and providing them with no sunlight appears to cause diseases. Perhaps when we eat diseased malnourished animals they will cause us to have health problems too. You are what you eat!

7. PROTEIN LEAVES AN ACID RESIDUE IN OUR BODIES.

We need to maintain a proper ratio of acid to alkaline in our bodies. An overly acid or basic condition in our bodies

[1] "Diet and Stress and Vascular Disease," *Journal of the American Medical Association*, 3 June 1961, p. 806.

2." *Diet for A New America,*" By John Robbins, 1987

may set up the conditions for disease. Note that fruits and vegetables are alkaline when ripe while animal foods and nuts are more acid.

When more protein is consumed than the body can process, the blood will become toxic from the excessive amount of nitrogen in the blood.

"Many people feel more energetic after eating high protein foods. This is because the chemical composition of uric acid is much like that of caffeine. What you're feeling is not increased energy, but chemical stimulation."[1]

8. ANIMAL PROTEIN IS ADDICTIVE.

When I tried to go off animal protein in order to become a vegetarian, I went into a withdrawal much like a drug addict experiences. Initially I craved animal protein terribly and would have to eat it when I was detoxifying too rapidly. This would completely stop my healing crisis and give me an artificial stimulation.

"Concentrated foods such as starch, meat, cheese, and sugar cause the most excitement and are the most addicting."[2]

Now after establishing my vegetarian diet, I find I have no desire to eat animal food. Eating animal food looks as appealing as eating a rock.

9. ENERGY EXCHANGE.

The body works very hard digesting animal protein. Our bodies should not have to digest food all day long; this weakens the body, not giving it time to repair and rebuild itself. Fruits and vegetables are easily digested, taking about 2-4 hours to replenish the enzymes to the cells.

10. NATURE INTENDED A VEGETARIAN DIET FOR US.

All animals have the anatomy and physiology for getting and utilizing the kinds of food that nature intended for them, and on which they will survive best.

---

[1] D. Eugene Briggs, PhD, *Your Lymph System, the Health Key.*

[2] Jeffrey Mannix, *Food Combining*, pp. 7, 8

11. KILLING SOULS IS NOT OUR RIGHT.

We have no right to shorten animals' life spans and to torture them. I was telling my husband how good it felt not to have to eat from dead souls (animals) any more. He said that animals have no souls. "But, John," I said, "It's right in the Bible, Genesis, 1:22, 'and to every beast of the earth and to every fowl of the air, and to every thing that creepeth upon the earth, wherein there is a living soul, I have given every green herb for food'."

Animals and fowl are being debeaked alive, put in dark pens with no sunshine, no room to even walk or sit, drugged, and tortured and with no mother nor father to nest with and, then, killed as if they are just soulless, money-making objects.

12. THE CONSUMPTION OF ANIMAL PRODUCTS IS VERY WASTEFUL.

According to information from the USDA, over 90% of the grain produced in America is used for feeding livestock. This grain could be used for human consumption, providing higher quality protein and conserving land, energy, and resources.

"For every 16 pounds of grain and soy fed to beef cattle in the United States, we only get 1 pound back in meat on our plates."[1]

To give you some basis for comparison, 16 pounds of grain has twenty-one times more calories and eight times more protein—but only three times more fat—than a pound of hamburger.

13. THE FARMING OF ANIMALS USES MUCH MORE WATER THAN GROWING VEGETABLES.

We are in a crisis with water and need to conserve. "I realized that the water used to produce just 10 pounds of steak equals the household consumption of my family for the entire year."[2]

---

[1] Frances Moore Lappe, *Diet for a Small Planet,* pp. 69, 84, 169.
[2] Ibid.

Animal chart 1

THE CARNAVORA	THE OMNIVORA	THE HERBIVORA	THE ANTHROPOID APES	HUMANS
Zonary placenta	Placenta non-deciduate	Placenta non-deciduate	Discoidal placenta	Discoidal placenta
Four footed	Four footed	Four footed	Two hands and two feet	Two hands and two feet
Have paws and claws	Have hooves	Have hooves (cloven)	Flat nails	Flat nails
Go on all fours	Go on all fours	Go on all fours	Upright or semi-upright	Walk upright
Have tails	Have tails	Have tails	Without tails	Without tails
Eyes look sideways	Eyes look sideways	Eyes look sideways	Eyes look forward	Eyes look forward
Skin with pores	Skin with pores	Skin with pores	Millions of pores	Million of pores
Slightly developed incisor teeth	Very small developed incisor teeth	Grazing animal; no upper incisors. Cartilage pad	Well-developed incisor teeth	Well-developed incisor teeth
Pointed molar teeth	Molar teeth in folds	Molar teeth in folds	Blunt molar teeth	Blunt molar teeth
* Dental formula	Dental formula	Dental formula	Dental formula	Dental formula
5to8/1/6/1/5to8 (upper)	8/1/2or3/1/8	6/0/0/6	8/11/4/1/5	5/1/4/1/5
5to8/1/6/1/5to8 (lower)	8/1/2or3/1/8	6/1/6/1/6	8/11/4/1/5	5/1/4/1/5

Animal chart 2

THE CARNAVORA	THE OMNIVORA	THE HERBIVORA	THE ANTHROPOID APES	HUMANS
Small salivary glands	Well-developed Salivary glands	Well-developed salivary glands	Well-developed salivary glands	Well-developed salivary glands
Acid reaction of saliva and urine	Acid reaction of saliva and urine	Acid reaction of saliva and urine	Acid reaction of saliva and urine	Acid reaction of saliva and urine
Rasping tongue	Smooth tongue	Smooth tongue	Smooth tongue	Smooth tongue
Teats on abdomen	Teats on abdomen	Teats on abdomen	Mammary glands located on chest	Mammary glands located on chest
Stomach simple and roundish	Stomach simple and roundish; large cul-de-sac	Ruminant stomach is in four compartments	Stomach with duodenum (as second stomach)	Stomach with duodenum (as second stomach)
Intestinal canal 3 times length of body	Intestinal canal 10 times length of body	Intestinal length varies by species; usually 10 times length of body	Intestinal canal 12 times length of body (torso)	Intestinal canal 12 times length of body (torso)
Colon smooth	Intestinal canal smooth and convoluted	Intestinal canal smooth and convoluted	Colon convoluted	Colon convoluted
Lives on flesh-foods	Lives on flesh-foods carrion or offal, and plants	Lives on grass, herbs, plant items	Normal diet vegetarian	Should live on totally vegetarian diet
*Looking across entire mouth molars/canines/ incisors/molars				

From *The Juniour Hygenists*

14. ANIMAL WASTE (FECES AND URINE) IS POLLUTING THE RIVERS AND WATER SYSTEMS.

Because of their large size, animals produce three times more waste than humans. The manure is high in ammonia and nitrates which, if dumped into our rivers or leached into our water supplies, can create too high nitrate levels. High nitrate levels in our bodies can cause brain damage.

7

ENZYMES

Lack of knowledge of the importance of enzymes in our diet may be the most glaring error of the food industry. Currently people are concerned about their fiber intake, knowing that it is extremely important to eat fiber to help keep the colon clean. This is true, but eating fiber is not as important as eating live enzymes. One day, the whole world will recognize enzyme nutrition as one of the best ways to strengthen the immune system. When this happens, the food industry will write the enzyme content on every package and how the food is processed to keep enzymes alive.

WHAT ARE ENZYMES?

"Enzymes are believed to have played key roles in the processes that led to the formation of life on this planet and to the gradual evolution into forms that now occupy the earth. Enzymes are the molecular activators, the overseers, the regulators, the universal agents of life. Enzymes are needed for every chemical action and reaction in the body. Our organs' tissues and cells are all run by metabolic enzymes. Minerals, vitamins, and hormones need enzymes to be present in order to do their work properly. Enzymes are the labor force of the body".[1]

Our bodies are made up of billions upon trillions of cells. Enzymes activate these cells. Every second 7 million cells are dying, and every second 7 million new cells are being formed. A single drop of blood contains about forty billion cells.

---

[1] David M. Locke, *Enzymes, The Agents of Life*, p.2

Every different kind of cell has its own special group of enzymes to make them function.

Enzymes are the key to health. Enzymes bring the nutrients into the cells, and enzymes flush out the waste. Enzymes are the activators of every amino acid chain; every movement of your body is started by enzymes. As an aid in digestion, saliva contains enzymes to begin breaking down the food when it enters our mouths.

Enzymes are found in raw food only. When you cook your food, whether in a microwave oven, a gas stove or an electric stove, this vital ingredient is destroyed.

David M. Locke says, "To get enzymes from food, one must eat raw food. All life, whether plant or animal, requires the presence of enzymes to keep it going; therefore, all plant and animal food in raw state has them....The remarkable thing about the eventual bankruptcy of the enzyme account is that it can proceed quite painlessly, without immediate symptoms."

The mere touch of heat destroys the enzymes. They do not tolerate any heat at all. They are different from vitamins in this respect. Pasteurization also destroys the life force in them, even though much less heat is used than in cooking. If water is hot enough to feel uncomfortable to the hand, it will injure enzymes in food.

Dr. Edward Howell, author of *Enzyme Nutrition,* says "...until I found out how ultra sensitive enzymes are to heat, I did not realize that the human race had been trying to get along without a whole category of food ingredients since cooking began. Therefore, instead of 1932 being an era representing a pinnacle in nutritional knowledge, I have come to regard it as the dark ages of nutrition."

In *The Chemicals of Life, Enzymes and Hormones,* Isaac Asimov states, "Heat is very hard on proteins. Molecules vibrate as a result of heat. The higher the temperature, the harder they vibrate. It doesn't take much vibration to shake loose the complicated structure of a globular protein. And when we say heat, we can't mean a match flame. We don't even mean boiling water. An ordinary warm summer day is hot enough to destroy an enzyme. In order to keep enzyme solution alive when studied, it must be frozen solid. This is how fragile they are."

Francis Pottenger, Jr., MD gives, in his *Pottenger's Cats, a Study in Nutrition,* the results of a 10-year diet study of 600 cats. The results showed the destructive effects of cooked foods—simply put, cats fed a raw diet were healthier and lived longer than cats fed a cooked diet. After Dr. Pottenger studied several generations of cats, he concluded that "An optimum diet refers to a diet of raw food including raw meat, raw milk and cod liver oil. A deficient diet refers to a diet including one or more cooked meats plus cod liver oil."

FIRST GENERATION DIET-DEFICIENT CATS—

"Heart problems; nearsightedness, farsightedness; under activity of the thyroid or inflammation of the thyroid gland; infection of the kidney, of the liver, of the testes, of the ovaries; arthritis, inflammation of the joints; inflammation of the nervous system with paralysis and meningitis."

SECOND GENERATION DIET-DEFICIENT CATS—

"These cats are the kittens born to females at the first deficient generation. All symptoms have become progressively worse from one generation to the next. Much more irritable, dangerous to handle, sex interest is slack or perverted, role reversal, allergies and skin lesions. Such sexual deviations are not observed among the raw food cats."

"Abortion in pregnant females is common, running about 25 percent in the first deficient generation to about 70 percent in the second generation. Deliveries are generally difficult with many females dying in labor. The mortality rate of the kittens also is high as the kittens are either born dead or are born too frail to nurse."

THIRD GENERATION DIET-DEFICIENT CATS—

These cats are the kittens born to females of the second generation eating a deficient diet.

"There are never more than three generations of deficient cats because of the third generation's inability to produce healthy, viable offspring."

"By the time the third deficient generation is born, the cats are so bankrupt that none survive beyond the sixth month of life, thereby terminating the strain."

OPTIMUM-DIET CATS—

"The cats fed a diet of 2/3 raw meat, 1/3 raw milk and cod liver oil show striking uniformity in their sizes and their skeletal developments. From generation to generation they maintain a regular, broad fare with prominent maler and orbital arches, adequate nasal cavities, broad dental arches and regular dentition. The configuration of the female skull is different from the male skull and each sex maintains its distinct anatomical features. The membranes are firm and of good, pink color with no evidence of infection or degenerative change."

Dr. Pottenger went on to study plants fertilized by manure from the cats fed raw foods and manure from cats fed cooked foods. He took two separate grounds and fertilized each. The plants with the raw food manure grew excellently. The plants with the cooked food manure grew terribly. This shows the effects of deficient soil, which causes weak plants or animals and weak, sickly humans.

Enzymes are the missing link in health. In the book *Roger's Recovery from Aids*, Bob Owens writes how Roger and he figured out the effect on health between a cooked diet and a high live enzyme diet. This gave Roger the choice between dying from AIDS or living with a new live foods diet. The answer is so simple, a matter of fact. Yet even the high enzyme diet may not be easy enough for most of us. People seem to prefer miracles or magic cures and are reluctant to change their dietary habits. They are not going to get it by wishful thinking. It takes perseverance and discipline to be able to stay on a live foods diet. We are constantly bombarded with literature for non-optimum food that's bad for us. We are told to feed our children the food because they will love it, it tastes good, and it's fun. This makes it hard for people to stay on a raw diet. The so called nutritional experts tell us it is okay to eat this way. Also, you have to deal with junk food at social gatherings and with family members who eat potato chips, chicken, cookies, cake, steak...in front of you, constantly telling you how good this food is for you. When we are conditioned all our life to eat a certain way it becomes a recognized pattern that feels right. It reminds us of home, mom, dad, and love.

I have read of people who, when dying of cancer, learn the meaning of a live enzyme diet. When they adopt the live diet they get healthier and are able to fight the cancer. In *How I Conquered Cancer Naturally,* Eydie Mae Koenig writes, "We learned a lot about the preparation and combining of raw foods, enzymes in 'live' food (anything raw, seeds, nuts, etc.) how cooking destroys enzymes (important to cancer people because they have a digestive problem, especially with protein, and enzymes are needed in order to digest food)."

"When there are no food enzymes in the food you eat to predigest it, your pancreas must enlarge to give out more internal enzymes to do the job....This is precisely the situation that intractable ailments such as cancer, hypertension, heart disease, and arthritis need to get going."

Ann Wigmore in her book *The Hippocrates Diet* says, "The most thrilling experience I can recall was to see cancer cells taken from a human body and thriving on cooked food but unable to survive on the same food when its was uncooked."

Susan Jorg writes in *Healthful Living Magazine* [Texas]—

1. Raw foods are better quality, therefore you eat less to satisfy your nutritional needs. The heat of cooking depletes vitamins, damages proteins and fats, and destroys enzymes which benefit digestion. As your percentage of raw foods increases, you feel satisfied and have more energy on smaller meals because raw food has the best balance of water, nutrients, and fiber to meet your body's needs.

2. Raw foods have more flavor than cooked foods so there is no need to add salt, sugar, spices, or other condiments that can irritate your digestive system or overstimulate other organs.

3. Raw foods take very little preparation so you spend less time in the kitchen. Even a child of 5 or 6 can prepare most items for breakfast, lunch or dinner. This gives children a sense of self- esteem and independence, not to mention the break it gives Mom or Dad.

4. When you are eating raw, there's little chance of burns, unless you're in the middle of a forest fire or out in the sun too long. Just think! NO burns to tongues, the roof of your mouth, nor fingers, and many fewer house fires.

5. Cleaning up after a raw meal is a snap. No baked-on oils or crusty messes. Any inedible parts go directly to the compost pile.

6. Eating a diet of raw foods may reverse or stop the advance of many chronic diseases, including heart disease and cancer. Cooking creates highly reactive chemicals called free radicals. These may be a major cause of cancer. When you lower the number of free radicals your cells are bombarded with, you lower your risk of cancer.

7. A raw food diet can protect you from acute diseases such as colds, flu, measles, etc. Raw foods maintain a healthy body and a healthy body will not become diseased.

8. As long as you combine raw food properly according to the rules of Natural Hygiene, you will soon reach a level where you no longer suffer from heartburn, gas, indigestion, or constipation.

9. It is environmentally sound. With humanity on a diet of raw foods, the food industry would close up shop and take up organic gardening. This would save us enormous amounts of natural resources used to produce power for these industries. Nuclear power would be clearly unnecessary. And think of how many trees and oil reserves could be saved without the need for the paper and plastics used in packaging our processed foods. There would also be less carbon dioxide released into the atmosphere when all the cooking stopped and more oxygen produced from all the new orchards and gardens, thus helping to reverse the Greenhouse Effect.

10. Eating raw saves you money on food, vitamins, pots and pans, appliances, doctor bills, drugs, and health insurance.

I have been trying to follow a complete raw food diet for the past 6 years. So far I have been able to reach a 95% raw foods diet. I feel fantastic when eating this way.

When I found out how important a raw diet was, I immediately tried to change my diet but found I could not. My stomach would not digest raw foods in the beginning because it was sluggish and lazy. So I started with one small piece of raw carrot the first week and slowly kept adding more the following weeks. I learned that if I ate lots of high enzyme fruits such as papaya and pineapple (tropical fruit is high in enzymes) they would help build up my enzyme pool and make raw vegetables slip nicely through my stomach. Fruits have a much higher enzyme count then vegetables.

Dr. L. M. Abramowski says "The milk of every animal in its natural state represents the most vitalizing food for its own offspring but when thoroughly cooked, its food-value becomes negative; it destroys life instead of sustaining it."

Think of all our babies being fed dead formulas and dead bottled baby foods. This generation is the first to experience a completely dead diet at birth. Prior to our modern life, mothers themselves chewed the food before feeding it to the baby. Doing so allowed a mother to ease their baby's digestion process by breaking down the food with enzymes in her own saliva. Today everything is so fast paced it's depressing to consider what problems the next generation might suffer as a result of the dead food diet.

The Food and Drug Administration appears to have no idea that enzymes are the missing link to radiant health since they never advocate eating live foods. In fact they stress the opposite. The FDA Consumer Report dated October 1990, reads "And the labeling of the Barley Green power was false in suggesting that cooking food is responsible for a deficiency in the quality of the daily diet and that conventional foods and diets represent the most serious threat to good health." Why don't they initiate studies on the benefits of live foods before making such uninformed statements?

FOOD COMBINING

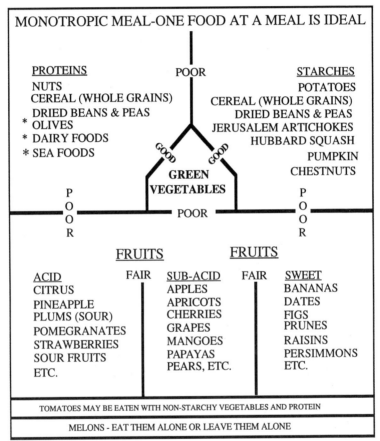

MONOTROPIC MEAL-ONE FOOD AT A MEAL IS IDEAL

PROTEINS
NUTS
CEREAL (WHOLE GRAINS)
DRIED BEANS & PEAS
* OLIVES
* DAIRY FOODS
* SEA FOODS

POOR

STARCHES
POTATOES
CEREAL (WHOLE GRAINS)
DRIED BEANS & PEAS
JERUSALEM ARTICHOKES
HUBBARD SQUASH
PUMPKIN
CHESTNUTS

GOOD GOOD

GREEN
VEGETABLES

POOR

POOR POOR

FRUITS FRUITS

ACID FAIR SUB-ACID FAIR SWEET
CITRUS APPLES BANANAS
PINEAPPLE APRICOTS DATES
PLUMS (SOUR) CHERRIES FIGS
POMEGRANATES GRAPES PRUNES
STRAWBERRIES MANGOES RAISINS
SOUR FRUITS PAPAYAS PERSIMMONS
ETC. PEARS, ETC. ETC.

TOMATOES MAY BE EATEN WITH NON-STARCHY VEGETABLES AND PROTEIN

MELONS - EAT THEM ALONE OR LEAVE THEM ALONE

*THESE SUBSTANCES ARE NOT RECOMMENDED BUT ARE INCLUDED FOR CLARITY
Copyright by Shangri La Natural Health Resort at Bonita Springs, Florida 3392

8

FOOD COMBINING

When I learned about food combining, I was deeply impressed. And when I began applying the rules my indigestion, gassiness, and sluggishness disappeared. Food combining even now seems miraculous.

T.C. Fry in his book, *Correct Food Combining for Easy Digestion and Wonderful Health*, writes:

> When I was a conventional eater I had antacid pills in my pockets, my desk drawer, on my night stand, in my auto and at other strategic points. Most of my meals were attended by violent and distressing heartburn, foul and embarrassing gas emissions and bad breath. Little did I realize that my mode of eating was the cause of my digestive problems.
>
> As a national testimonial to our chronic indigestion, there is a multi-million dollar antacid industry in this country. Tums, Rolaids, Alka Seltzer and numerous other preparations sell by the carload—over 100 billion doses a year are reportedly taken.

Eating foods that are hard to digest can cause stress on the body in the following ways.

1. Wastes body energy
2. Weakens immune system by causing high amounts of bacteria to flood the body.
3. Heartburn
4. Headache or Backache
5. Weakness or fatigue
6. Gas
7. Bad Breath
8. Disease
9. Obesity
10. Constipation or Diarrhea

Food combining refers to the best combinations of foods to eat at the same meal. The reason for food combining is very simple. Foods of different characteristics require different body enzymes and stomach conditions for digestion.

"It takes energy to eliminate, and the elimination cycle is of extreme importance. The body cannot eliminate toxic waste without your cooperation. The way we must assist the body is to supply it with readily available energy on a steady basis. This is the answer to being healthy and trim."[1]

The digestion of the food takes more energy than any other function of the body, so this is a great place to free up energy.

Too many food combinations create undigested foods (body toxins) which are stored in the fat cells. The biggest no-no is steak (protein) and potato (starch) eaten together. The two go down into the stomach and the body keeps kicking out different digestive juices which overwork the stomach. This may be the start of indigestion or heartburn. Then by peristaltic action of the intestines, the undigested food moves down into the intestines to set up the possibility of colon problems. Now the protein and carbohydrate have completely fermented allowing rotting foul-smelling bacteria to flourish throughout the body.

Tests have demonstrated that undigested starch and protein may be found in the bowels of people who do wrong food combining.

People with Candida or other illnesses may greatly benefit from food combining because Candida seems to be an overgrowth of yeast in the intestines. If no undigested food particles reach the intestines, there is nothing for the yeast to grow on, thereby eliminating the problem. This is analogous to a clean kitchen. For example, if crumbs were left on the kitchen floor, bugs would find them and happily flourish. Keep the kitchen clean, the bugs stay away. Isn't it the same in our intestines?

What we want is for our food to pass through our bodies and be digested in three hours or less with no heartburn or gas. Proper food combining achieves this goal.

---

[1] Harvey Diamond, *Fit for Life*.

HOW IS FOOD COMBINING DONE?

This is done by only eating starches (potatoes, rice, beans, wheat, oats...) with green vegetables at one meal and eating proteins with vegetables at another. That is, you have a choice of eating either protein and greens together or starch and greens together but never protein and starch at the same meal.

Fruit is divided into three groups: Acid—oranges, grapefruit, lemon; Subacid—apple, pear; Sweet—banana, dates. By looking at the food combining chart on page 60 you can see what goes together. Fruit is never eaten with starches and acid and sweet should never be eaten together.

I also think it depends on how healthy one's digestive system is. It appears that people with strong digestion have more enzymes to break down food and become healthier because of this. Some healthy individuals seem to be able to digest foods in all food combinations. Also it may be that an all raw food diet with its abundant supply of enzymes may allow you to not be so strict about food combining.

I, personally, have found food combining to be a life saver. I eat many foods in what is called a mono diet. This means at any one meal I only allow myself one kind of food, for instance, only apples or only bananas. I find food easier to digest this way. I have found my body tells me how much to eat at one sitting. If I eat too much I become tired after the meal. Listen to your body. For example, three bananas are too much for me to eat at one meal. Also, noting the time I eat a food has helped me focus on how long it takes to digest, say, an apple. If I wait two hours before eating another meal, that meal is allowed to reach deep down into my colon before a new meal is started. We also need to be aware that even if the food has left the stomach, it does not mean it has been fully digested. It must reach the lower bowels before it is time to eat again.

9

SLOW CHANGE

The first thing to learn about changing to a vegetarian diet, or at least to a better diet, is to make the change slowly. I learned about this the hard way. Our bodies have been sustained for years by all the wrong materials (hot dogs, hamburgers, steak, chicken, french fries, coke, ice cream, cookies, sugars, etc.). We have to get rid of the byproducts of these long years of bad eating. When we do this we will shed lots of unwanted toxic cells. This process will cause us discomfort and in the beginning could make us extremely frail and weak. When older people or very sickly people try to change to a better diet, they will find that it is very difficult because their organs are in a weak and sluggish condition. The new raw foods hurt their stomach, and may possibly cause an irritable bowel or a slight shaky feeling. They should go though a transitional diet first, which allows their toxins to be removed gradually and their digestion systems to strengthen slowly. They can start by eating a small piece of raw food at each meal and by adding live juices and fresh fruit to their diet.

When I changed my diet too quickly, it was quite unpleasant. The raw foods would come though my bowels undigested and irritate the lining of my colon. To prevent this, I cooked my food until it was mush. The longer I cooked the vegetables, the easier they seemed to digest. Little by little, I added the raw foods, giving my body time to strengthen and entirely digest the raw foods. Only in this way was I able to receive the full benefit of the superior raw foods. It took me six months to improve to a condition where I could eat a raw diet.

When my husband and I began an all raw foods diet, we lost fat and appeared to be anorexic. We even lost fat from our rears and it hurt when we sat down. We received much verbal abuse from our friends who continued telling us that what we were doing was wrong. It took me over 18 months to get my body fat back and my weight (which had dropped to 88 pounds) back to a normal 105. My husband lost over 60 pounds from his overweight 270 pound body. He's now a perfect 215 on a 6'7" frame and is very happy about this. He was able to quit smoking, quit drinking coffee, change to vegetarian diet (no animal foods), add whole herb foods, and stick to a diet of 80 percent raw foods and 20 percent cooked. His health improved—hay fever disappeared, and an infection in his eye (he suffered with iritis for 3 years) was gone. He was happier, and did not need as much sleep. This didn't happen overnight and he went through many cleanses to reach this improved state.

You will hear some people say, "Oh, I tried all that raw food and it didn't work for me." You have to be patient and find your balance. Everybody and every body is different. Your digestion might not be ready to digest raw food if it is too weak and you may lack the enzymes required for good digestion. Our bodies need lots of enzymes to break down the raw vegetables, so don't forget to eat lots of fruit which naturally contain high amounts of enzymes.

I discovered that many special diets limit fruit, Macrobiotic and Candida-control diets in particular. Advocates for both say fruit, although high in protein, carbohydrates, water, oils, and minerals, contains too much sugar. I found through my own experimentation that they are wrong, that fruit is one of the best foods for people like myself who suffer from Candida. The much feared fruit sugar is no problem because it is predigested in our mouths and none is leftover for bacteria to grow on.

Be aware that there are three different categories of fruit: sweet, acid, and alkaline. Try to eat from all categories to ensure a complete balanced diet.

Because of poor advice, I did not eat fruit for 7 years. I agreed with the advice because every time I tried to eat fruit I became ill with a spastic colon. I didn't know at that time this happened because fruit contained a high amount of enzymes and that the enzymes were cleansing the waste from my body cells and regenerating them into better ones. You need to understand regeneration to realize how fruit does its cleaning—causing some irritation in the beginning.

However, Macrobiotic and the Candida diet are good transitional diets on the way to the perfect raw food diet.

It was hard work to figure out what type of food is needed, how much to eat at one sitting, how long does digestion take, and how much chewing is enough to ensure complete digestion. My thoughts were: will the meal supply adequate enzymes and is there a need for more high chlorophyll green foods (romaine lettuce, wheat grass, broccoli, etc.)? The answer slowly came and was surprisingly simple: the key to health is to get our nutritional needs from natural foods and to eat them with as little processing as possible.

I read about mothers changing their children's diet to a vegetarian one and then finding that their children became anemic. They knew that even though meat is a source of iron, red foods (watermelon, beets, etc.) contain far more usable iron for us. The vegetarian diet was correct, but the problem was that they had fed their children a cooked and high dairy diet. That is what caused them to be malnourished. If they had done more research and realized that the children should be fed a balanced diet of raw plants, herbs, fruits, nuts, and seeds this would not have happened. My daughter has been a vegetarian for three years and is far healthier than she was before the change in diet. She used to see the doctor monthly because of chronic ear infections and bronchitis. Now she has no problems and has not been to a doctor for over five years.

I called a health organization to ask what they thought of changing one's diet to a raw food diet? I was told, "Not every one can do a completely raw diet. It is the best diet, but most people can do well on an 80 percent raw foods and 20 percent cooked diet. Eating cooked grains and vegetables seems to help some people immediately put weight back on. Raw fiber is difficult for some people's digestion systems to handle and heating the food appears to aid in breaking the fibrous part down to make vitamins more available. Cooking does appear to make some of the food components dangerous."

Now that you are aware of these new ideas on whole raw foods, you might want to try testing them. If you do, first determine if foods control you. You probably are thinking, no way. I control what I eat, not the other way around. Try this. Eat a sweet chocolate doughnut. When you're through, feel the sour aftertaste in your mouth. Compare this to eating one orange, notice the sparkling clean taste an orange leaves behind. Next, compare the amount of food that can be eaten cooked to the amount you can eat raw. You may be able to eat a head of broccoli if it is cooked, but if it were raw your jaw would probably hurt (natural reaction) after a while of chewing and the pain would prevent you from over eating.

Interestingly, I found the easier it is to chew raw foods the easier it is to digest them. Notice the way a papaya dissolves in you mouth compared to a piece of cabbage. The easily chewed raw food has more enzymes.

Realize, too, that if there is a sour coating on your teeth there is probably also one on your intestines. Mucus in the throat indicates a mucus coating in the intestines as well; and a mucus coating in the intestines will cause malabsorption of nutrients. We all brush our teeth every day as if it's the only place grime gets stuck, what about the grime in our intestines!

There can be an improvement in our teeth when we change to a better diet. Our teeth can become sharper from a raw diet. Vegetables, nuts and seeds sharpen our teeth to help us digest our food better. On a cooked diet our teeth never get the chance to improve. They are dull from eating so much mushy food and dull teeth are one of the major reasons people can't eat raw.

My jaw realigned itself after I changed to a raw food diet. This was because my teeth realigned themselves naturally causing the T.M.J. to go away.

We buy cheap food not realizing we don't save money because we're still hungry when we finish eating. When we eat this food we lay a coating of mucus in our colons which prevents us from absorbing nutrients; we're still hungry. We eat more food because our body continues to starve for nutrients. But this is not true with a raw diet. You will eventually need to eat one meal a day because your body will work so well it will be satisfied and not hunger for nutrients.

I feel we all naturally know that this is the correct diet. We don't want to admit it, even to ourselves. We hide from the truth. We know processed food is inferior. Although we say we are the masters of nature, it's not true. Nature can shake us, storm us and drown us if need be. We must go back to nature and work in harmony with the environment. We must feed the earth so that the earth will take care of us. When we pollute the world, we pollute ourselves. When we strip the earth, we strip ourselves. When we follow the path of harmony with the universe of life, we become flowing full of truths, love and knowledge.

TABLE OF FOOD COMPOSITION

	Human Milk	Whole Milk
Measure	1 cup	1 cup
Weight (grams)	244	244
Calories	168	159
Carbohydrate (g)	16.96	11.4
Protein (g)	2.56	8.5
Fiber (g)	0	0
Saturated fat (g)	4.96	5.07
Unsaturated fat (g)	5.28	2.65
Total fat (g)	10.8	8.15
Cholesterol (mg)	32	33
Vitamin A (IU)	592	350
Vitamin B (mg)	.032	.093
Vitamin B_1 (mg)	.088	.395
Vitamin B_2 (mg)	.024	.102
Vitamin B_{12} (mg)	.112	.871
Biotin (mcg)	t	5
Folic Acid (mg)	.016	.012
Niacin (mg)	.44	.205
Pantothenic Acid (mg)	.552	.766
Vitamin C (mg)	12.32	2.29
Vitamin E (mg)	.552	.293
Sodium (mg)	40	120
Phosphorus (mg)	32	228
Potassium (mg)	128	351
Calcium (mg)	80	291
Iron (mg)	.08	.12
Magnesium (mg)	8	33
Copper (mg)	.12	.5
Manganese (mg)	t	.005
Selenium (mg)	0	3.17
Zinc	.40	.93

10

ENERGY EXCHANGE

Our bodies exchange energy with the outside world via the five senses. Eating food is one of the ways, for better or for worse, we do this. If we eat foods that are easy to digest we minimize the expenditure of body energy and have more energy to help the body function. When we eat hard to digest foods we use a lot of body energy because our digestion systems have to work hard and long to assimilate the foods, taking energy away from other body functions such as thinking, moving, and elimination. For instance, if we have a sick body then we need the most energy to fight the disease and eating difficult to digest foods may not be the best thing to do at this time.

Fruit is the easiest food to digest. In a properly functioning body it is predigested in the mouth leaving almost no work for the stomach. It is also the food highest in water content. The high water content is useful because our bodies are made of 80 percent water and we need a lot of water to function. This does not necessarily mean we should drink lots of water instead of eating. But it is best to get water from natural sources like fruit. Interestingly, if we eat a high water diet (raw foods) we probably will never be thirsty. In addition to the high water content, fruit has high enzyme content (tropical fruit has the highest amount of enzymes in a food) and can supply sugar to feed the brain and other body functions. Next to fruit, vegetables are an easy to digest food. Their water content is also high. After them come sprouted grains and beans, and then nuts and seeds. It appears that, if we use human mothers' milk as a guide, the more the food's nutrients differ from mothers' milk the harder the food is to digest (see chart on p. 68). Also, by examining foods in their whole form, you should be able to get an idea about the difficulty of the process of digesting them. For instance, by the time you get through just cracking the shells on nuts you could have eaten and digested an apple.

DIGESTION TIME OF FOOD—4 OZS (ON AVERAGE)

Fruit	1-2 hours
Vegetables	2-3 hours
Grains	3 hours
Nuts and Seeds	3-4 hours
Animal Products	5 or more hours

It appears that a simple diet may allow the body to work at its optimum condition. It could be that a mono diet is the best diet because the body can assimilate the nutrients easier due to the lesser confusion associated with eating one food at a time. Let's say you're making a cake. One recipe has five ingredients and the other calls for twenty ingredients. You don't feel like working hard so you decide to make the five ingredient cake. This will take you fifteen minutes. You know the other cake will take longer, say forty-five minutes, since there are more than three times as many ingredients to work with. The same is true for the body—the fewer ingredients you put in your mouth, the easier it is to digest them. Less time spent in digestion should give you more energy to do other things.

GENERAL GUIDE TO HOW DIET EFFECTS SLEEP

Diet	Sleep Required (hours)
Fasting (water or nothing)	2 to 4
Fruit only	4 to 6
Vegetables, fruit, nuts, and seeds	6 to 8
Meat, fruits, vegetables, and grains	8 to 10

The better you eat the more awake energy you have! I try to eat only three meals a day:

Breakfast	- One piece of fruit
Lunch	- Raw vegetables, sprouts, and herbs
Dinner	- Fruit (two of the same kind)

If I decide to snack, I eats nuts, seeds, and herbs I am seldom hungry and can go up until 3:00pm without eating, shaking or having a headache. I used to suffer from hypoglycemia on a cooked food diet. I have been on a raw food diet for six years. The first year I decreased my food consumption by one-half and have maintained this level since then. Yet, I have gained weight—ten pounds in the second year.

ROTATIONAL DIET

The Rotational Diet, requires a change of ingredients every day, thereby giving the body an abundance of different kinds of nutrients.

It is important to eat just fruits one day each week. Doing so gives the digestive system a rest because fruit permits the easiest energy exchange with the body. If you want to know how to identify foods that are in the fruit family understand that fruit is labeled "fruit" because of seeds inside; therefore, those foods that contain seeds such as cucumber, squash, and tomatoes are in the fruit family.

For example, a typical four day diet may look like this.

Day One	Day Two	Day Three	Day Four
Sweet Potato	Artichoke	Corn	Peas or Limas
Asparagus	Cabbage	Butternut Squash	Beets, Celery
Spinach	Kale	Spaghetti Squash	Turnips
String Beans	Broccoli	Yellow Squash	Avocado
Pear	Bananas	Green Squash	Orange
	Almonds	Apple	Carrots
		Squash Seeds	Lettuce
		Pumpkin Seeds	

FASTING

I believe that fasting is one of the best ways to maximize energy in the human body. Also, when the body is given no food to digest, it doesn't have to use up energy for digestion and can utilize it for healing our bodies.

The best time for the body to clean up debris is in the morning; therefore, this is an ideal time to fast so as not to interfere with this cleansing process. Don't forget that not eating between meals is another way to allow more energy for the body.

I eat at 9:00 A.M. (Breakfast), 12:30 P.M. (Lunch), and 5:00 P.M. (Dinner). If I happen to have digestion problems, such as gassiness or body odor, I stop eating breakfast.

On longer fasts, seven days or more, it is possible to see major health problems subsiding.

"Anyone experienced with fasting has seen great numbers of such instances of physical rejuvenation achieved by means of the fast. The mental improvements commonly match the physical improvements. Occasional restoration of hearing in ears that have been deaf for years, improved vision discarding glasses that have been worn for years (but rarely restoration of sight to blind eyes), increased acuteness of the senses of taste and smell, restoration of ability to sense delicate flavors, recovery of the sense of feeling in instances of sensory paralysis, stepped up vigor, increased mental powers, loss of weight, greatly increased functional vigor, with better digestion and better bowel action, clear sparkling eyes, clearing of the complexion with a restoration of youthful bloom, the disappearance of some of the finer lines of the face, reduced blood pressure, better heart action, reduction of enlarged prostate, sexual rejuvenation—these and many other evidences of rejuvenation are seen by everyone who has a wide experience with fasting.

"Fasting can bring about a virtual rebirth, a revitalization of the organism. As the fast progresses, all of the cells of the body undergo refinement and there is a removal from the protoplasm of the cells of stored foreign substances (metaplasmic materials) so that the cells become more youthful and function more efficiently.

"Some of these stored materials are highly toxic and have long remained in the fatty cells and in the cells of the connective tissues which have been appropriately termed the 'dumping ground of the body' to get them out of the circulation. Freeing the tissues of such materials renders the body more efficient as a physiologic mechanism. Besides the renovation that fasting enables the body to undergo, there is created a potential for better function which continues long after the fast has been broken."[1]

My friends who have fasted for seven days tell me that they felt better than ever while fasting. They said that after the first couple of days, there is no more hunger, but there is an increase of energy. Fasting should be done under the supervision of an expert.

[1] Herbert M. Shelton, *Fasting Can Save Your Life.*

I feel that there is a direct link between aging and cell wastes or chronic toxic saturation. When I started following a small meals, raw foods diet, with fasting in the morning, I literally had no odor under my arms; my breath was fresh, and the aging process seemed to regenerate with wrinkles smoothing out on my face.

For more than fifteen years, Professor C. M. Child, of the University of Chicago, did research on aging in animals. His results revealed that periodic fasting is generally conducive to rejuvenescence.

In certain species of insects, he found that with an abundance of food, insects pass through their whole life-history in three to four weeks, but when the food is greatly reduced or the insects are forced to fast, they may continue active and young for at least three years. His conclusion was that 'partial starvation' (fasting) inhibits senescence.

How long can a person fast? We are told not to miss a meal, when the truth may be that we can live long, long periods without food. This period may be up to three months, or even longer. It depends on whether body reserves are adequate to meet the nutritive requirements of the body's functioning tissues.

When one fasts, the bacteria are eaten up first, then the fat; it goes in an inverse order. Then the stored reserves are used before the functioning tissues of the brain, nerves, heart, and lungs.

"One must differentiate between fasting and starving. To fast is to abstain from food when one possesses adequate reserves to nourish their vital tissues; to starve is to abstain from food when reserves have been exhausted so that vital tissues are sacrificed."

In this day and age, a long fast can be quite dangerous because air pollution, water pollution, and pesticides in our food have contaminated our bodies and the planet. Our bodies are not made up of perfect nourishment and a delicate balance between health and over toxicity may be occurring. So, no matter how great you think your body is, if you are receiving too many toxins from the outside environment, that may make it impossible to fast for a long period. For example, I have heard that people are able to do long fasts in the mountains, but are unable to do them in our filthy cities. I have seen people fast for seven days and have seen their ability to fight disease strengthen. This, however, does not mean that their bodies were made up of perfect ingredients. I have seen these same people try to eat highly nourishing herb foods and yet they still have their bodies react (regeneration and detoxification through diet) with flu-like symptoms. This is because they still have organs made up of the wrong materials. Just because fasting gets rid of the dirt does not mean that fasting will rebuild your body with better nutrients. You still need whole raw foods, sunlight, and pure water to rebuild body organs with better tissues.

If our bodies were fed only correct nourishment, we would be without most diseases and our bodies could operate on a small amount of raw food. We are all aware that a loss of desire for food is one of the first symptoms of disease. We don't always listen to our bodies, but we should. When we lose our desire for eating, our body is asking us to temporarily relieve it from the hard work of digesting food. Animals too behave in the same way. The first thing animals do when they get ill, in nature, is to fast.

The first meal after a fast should be an easily digestible food like fruit.

CHEWING FOOD

The human body's stomach was designed to digest liquids and small particles immersed in the liquids, not whole particles of food. Our teeth are there to chew up food particles until they are liquefied. There have been many people who have strengthened their immune systems by just changing this one aspect of their life. They chew their food 100 times before it goes down their throat. Our brains are triggered to release particular enzymes when we chew food. When we eat a carrot, the brain will signal enzymes to produce saliva to digest this carrot. This action is not there when we swallow vitamins or food—there is no brain-enzyme connection. Liquefying food by chewing also frees up much energy for digesting.

Think about this. We spend a lot of energy cleaning plaque from our teeth, yet we don't consider doing anything about cleaning up our insides which may be filthy with mucus, and hard impacted feces. We think that if we don't see the dirt, it's not there. In his book, *Tissue Cleansing Through Bowel Management,* Bernard Jensen, DC Nutritionist, writes:

"I believe that when the bowel is underactive, toxic wastes are more likely to be absorbed through the bowel wall and into the bloodstream from which they become deposited in the tissues. If any eliminative system is underactive, more wastes are retained in the body. As toxins accumulate in the tissues, increasing degrees of cell destruction take place. The digestion becomes poor and partially digested material adds to the problem because the body cannot make good tissue out of half digested nutrients. Proper function is slowed in all body tissues in which toxins have settled. When anyone has reached the degenerative disease state, it is a sign that toxic settlements have taken the body over. This is the time to have to consider detoxification—the cleansing of the body tissues...I am convinced and truly believe that our problem begins more in the bowel than any other part of the body. The body depends on a clean bowel. The cleanliness of any tissue, i.e., kidney, stomach, brain, depends upon what is found in the bowel...The heavy mucus coating in the colon thickens and becomes a host for putrefaction. The blood capillaries to the colon begin to pick up the toxins, poisons and noxious debris as it seeps through the bowel wall...It is an indisputable fact that not only illness and old age, but even death is due to the accumulation of waste products of body chemistry and, on the other hand, to the inability of the body to replenish its cellular structures and organs with fresh vital nutrients. Therefore, immunity and freedom from disease can be had and old age and death can be deferred only as long as body wastes are kept at a minimum and fresh, vital material of the first order is supplied for growth and repair of the body."

We should all be able to eliminate the residue of each meal 15 to 18 hours after eating it. The diet should be high in raw whole foods because the raw food fibers help clean the colon.

BREATHING

I remember one of my relatives who, at the age of 23, had problems with his colon. He was under much stress while going to college, particularly at final exam times. An MD told him he was sick because his breathing was too shallow. She said he needed to breathe deeply in order to massage his lower colon. When he did, his colon problems vanished.

"Not only does breathing keep us alive, it also activates all body mechanics and aids in all of our body functions. The major function of the heart and lungs is to produce and bring oxygen-rich blood to all body tissues. As the tissues are nourished, the mechanics of breathing act as an internal organ massage as well. When you inhale, air is brought into the lungs, the diaphragm descends, the thoracic cavity expands, and the pressure in the abdomen is increased. Exhaling causes the diaphragm to contract into a dome shape and increases the pressure within the thoracic cavity. Exhaling also puts pressure on the blood vessels and lymph tubes so that the fluids move up toward the heart, aiding circulation as it hastens the elimination of waste. As deep breathing helps our heart and lungs to work more effectively it also brings about a deep sense of relaxation, focus, harmony, and center."(Written in the book *Self-Massage* by Monika Struna with Connie Church).

"It's obvious that breathing is one of the most important functions of the body. Without breath, in minutes we would die.

"Man may exist some time without eating; a shorter time without drinking, but without breathing his existence may be measured by a few minutes...And not only is man dependent upon breath for life, but he is largely dependent upon correct habits of breathing for continued vitality and freedom from disease. An intelligent control of our breathing power will lengthen our days upon earth by giving us increased vitality and powers of resistance and, on the other hand, unintelligent and careless breathing will tend to shorten our days, by decreasing our vitality and laying us open to disease...Mans' mental power, happiness, self-control, clear-sightedness, morals, and even his spiritual growth may be increased by an understanding of the 'Science of Breath'...It is estimated that in a single day of twenty-four hours, 35,000 pints of blood traverse the capillaries of the lungs, the blood corpuscles passing in single file and being exposed to the oxygen of the air on both of their surfaces...A little reflection will show the inevitable importance of correct breathing. If the blood is not fully purified by the regenerative process of the lungs, it returns to the arteries in an abnormal state, insufficiently purified and imperfectly cleansed of the impurities which it took up on its return journey. These impurities, if returned to the system, will certainly manifest in some form of disease, either in a form of blood disease or some disease resulting from impaired functioning of some insufficiently nourished organ or tissue.

"The organs of respiration have their only protective apparatus, filter, or dust-catcher, in the nostrils. When the breath is taken through the mouth, there is nothing from mouth to lungs to strain the air, or to catch the dust and other foreign matter in the air."[1]

We go through all our life without anyone ever telling us the importance of breathing correctly. A simple thing such as breathing through your nose can help keep bacteria from coming into the body, thus making for one of the best things mothers can teach their children on how to fight against colds.

CALORIES

In the book *Food First,* the second book written after *Diet for a Small Planet,* Frances Moore Lappé and Joseph Collins write:

"Even now, with resources grossly under-used, Bangladesh grows enough in grain alone to provide everyone in the country with at least 2600 calories a day. Yet, according to nutrition surveys, over half of the families in Bangladesh daily consume less than 1500 calories per person, the minimum survival level. Two-thirds of the population suffer from protein and vitamin deficiencies."

The book is written to help diagnose the cause of hunger. The authors say that hunger is a people-made problem. "Hunger exists in the face of abundance—therein lies the outrage." Really the problem is a lack of knowledge.

A person should be able to live well on 1500 calories or less a day if the calories come from high quality foods. High enzyme foods that are nutritionally close to mothers' milk could supply fewer than 1500 calories but still be nutritionally adequate.

---

[1] Yogi Ramcharaka, *Science of Breath*, pp. 8, 15, 28.

A woman called me and said, "My doctor put me on a special diet to lose weight. I've been on this diet for a year. It is lettuce, cucumber, and celery. I've lost a lot of weight, but I get terrible food cravings, then I binge on everything. What do you think of these foods—am I getting enough protein?" My answer—You are getting two to three times the amount of protein that mothers' milk would supply, but protein is not the sole concern of eating. Your body needs to intake different nutrients to feed different parts of the body. Eating different colored foods can be a good way to ensure you're feeding every part of your body. All foods have their own special enzymes, minerals, amino acids, and carbohydrates. If you are not satisfied, usually this means you are missing a nutrient and your body is searching for it. By rotating the color of foods you may feel fewer cravings.

11

TOXINS

My father, age 60, is 5 foot 8 inches, weighs 155-pounds, has jet black hair, and is very visibly fit. He runs five miles each exercise period and does this four times a week. Because of his desire to help me regain my health, he began studying about diet. He succeeded in helping me, but found that for his own health he needed to change his diet from the standard American one supplemented with vitamins to a vegetarian diet which included whole food herbs. After doing this he told me that he felt better, saw colors better, had more energy, and felt an increase in internal peacefulness.

He continues to study and attends as many lectures as he can on holistic health. He and my mother have brought me information (tapes and papers) about lectures they have attended in California. One tape was very pertinent. I had been studying Dr. Max Gerson's book on cancer therapy, noting his diet was very high in fruits and vegetables, when much to my surprise my father sent me a taped lecture by Dr. Gerson's daughter, Charlotte Gerson. She was speaking in San Diego and he had gone to her lecture. I listened to her tape and agreed she is right on target.

Charlotte Gerson said, on November 2, 1989, "The Gerson therapy is healing, getting to the basic, underlying problems. Why are people ill? Why is the body not functioning? The problem is twofold: we are lacking the proper nutrients and we are too toxic. Actually, the body is starving, and at the same time the body is poisoned with all the toxic things that go into the food we eat, the air we breathe, and the water we drink or bathe in.

"It's definitely a dual problem—deficiency and toxicity. All disease, basically, falls in this category. In all of them, I have not found a single condition that is not based on deficiency and/or toxicity."

Now, let's start from the beginning. Dr. Gerson was a trained physician. Just as any other doctor, he attended medical school and learned that each disease has a diagnosis and that each disease has a drug or specific treatment. Chronic diseases, by definition, are deteriorating conditions of aging, and are not curable. If you think that when you have arthritis or when you have diabetes or high blood pressure, and you go to the doctor, he will cure you—NO WAY! There are no cures for chronic disease with orthodox medicine, by definition.

Dr. Gerson, at the age of 25, had severe migraine headaches to the point where he was throwing up. He went to his colleagues for help. The doctors told him that there was no cure, but, maybe, by the time you are 55, you will feel better. Dr. Gerson said, "I don't want to wait—I can't live this way." He felt that he had to research nutrition. He looked at the animals and found that our closest physiological relatives ate fruits, greens, nuts, and seeds. He started on apples, eating only apples (apple juice, apples cooked, raw apples), and found he felt better. He slowly added other foods back into his diet to see if he could handle them. If a food did not agree with him, he had a headache within twenty minutes. He also found that by eating lots of fruits and vegetables other problems he and his patients had also would go away.

ORGANIC FOODS

I have been eating organic foods for two years and have become aware of the considerable difference in nutritious quality between supermarket food and organically grown food. When I eat fruit and vegetables from the supermarket, my feet and hands become cold, I become tired, and I start developing a sore stomach and sore bladder; but when I eat organic produce, I feel great.

Consider this: if you want to buy a house, a car, or clothing, there are many choices and a noticeable difference in what money can buy. You can take your time to study the pros and cons of the item and weigh that off against the price. But if you want to buy produce, there is only one kind in the supermarket. There are no designer foods, limited or no labeling of produce, no telling us how it was grown or brochures or consumer organizations discussing and evaluating the nutritious quality of it. You almost always buy it with no knowledge of how it was raised, what country it came from, or if it was picked at the right time. What was its acid to alkaline balance? It seems that the foods are examined only for color or size, and certainly not for nutrients or minerals.

Could it be that the American people are selecting their foods from a low cost dime store? We spend so much money on vacations—a hundred dollars a day on average. We spend hundreds of thousands on a house, tens of thousands on cars, and thousands on diamond rings. But, to spend money on food for our bodies, we laugh at that thought. We say that organic food is too expensive. We are taught that only things on the outside are important, such as spending money on fashionable clothes. It costs so much to be ill. Right now health care in the USA costs nearly two billion dollars a day. Even with insurance, you might have to see a specialist whose costs are not covered. Not being able to work and enjoy life is also expensive. Please use a preventative approach and take care of yourself. Think before you eat. Your body and the quality of your life are much more important than clothes, cars, houses, jewelry, and furniture. Life starts with learning how to love ourselves, and then we can love others and love the planet.

If we keep polluting the outside world, we will be forced in the future to grow our food indoors. Do you think the plants will produce what they are capable of if they don't have natural sunlight and rainfall. Already, people like Ann Wigmore are growing plants indoors because of the pollution. The Ann Wigmore Foundation, in Boston, teaches how to do this for our survival. Ann feels we have reached the point where you can get more benefit from food grown fresh, indoors, because they contain more live enzymes, vitamins, and minerals.

So, save the coupons in the Sunday paper—20 cents here, 50 cents there. Cut them out and get reduced prices on dead food. We buy cheap food not realizing we don't save money because we're still hungry when we finish eating. In reality you are actually spending far more money on those foods with pesticides in them. Pesticides kill bugs. If they kill bugs, what do you think they do to a big bug (you)? They still kill, but much slower.

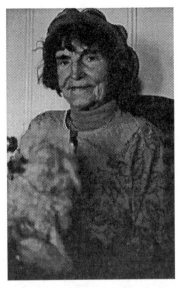

Here is Dr. Ann Wigmore in Backbay, Boston, at age 83. Up until her death in a fire on February 16, 1994, she had remained very active. She managed two Resorts and frequently held lectures throughout the world. She was completely devoted to a living foods lifestyle. At the age of 50, she found that she had cancer, motivating her to research wheat, grass, and sprouts, and develop indoor gardens and their relationship to disease. She has written many books including *Why Suffer?* and *The Hippocrates Diet.* Her books were published by Avery Publishing Group, Inc. in Wayne, NJ. More information is available through the Ann Wigmore Foundation, Boston, MA 01226. (617) 267-9424.

So you buy broccoli with pesticides on it. You say, "Oh, I can wash it off." Wrong. The pesticides are sprayed on top of the soil and, when watered, go into the roots of the plant, which, in turn, weakens the plant's resistance to bacteria and bugs. By giving the plant lots of nourishment, the plant strengthens and is able to fight bacteria and bugs. An organic farmer, speaking at a local Health Food Store, said, "I had to stop buying plants from commercial growers because their plants could not resist bugs, and, then, I had to come up with natural pesticides. I switched to organic starter plants and now I don't have the need for pesticides."

Now, you have eaten the $1.00 broccoli with chemicals. What if these chemicals eaten over many years weaken your immune system and cause you to develop cancer at age 35? You stop working. Your load is too heavy. Now, how many days did these chemicals, from one day's broccoli, take away from your life? Three days, maybe, which would equal, say, three days' pay, approximately $120.00. So, actually that broccoli cost you $120.00. You won't live as healthily, nor as long. But if you had eaten the organic, $1.50 broccoli, you might have added three days to your life, so you would have been paid $120.00 more. So, by eating organic broccoli, you would have made money, instead of a shortened life and net loss of $120.00.

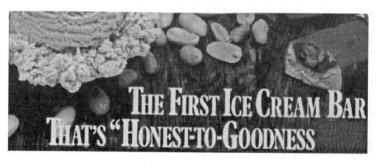

You read the ad and think when you eat this scrumptious candy bar, you're being good and kind to yourself. Not really, examine the list of ingredients. The amount of sugars, isolated chemicals, and cooked oils contained in one bar will significantly weaken your immune system. This, in turn, could create illness. So, in reality, this candy bar could cause loss of work and time, costing you from $100 to $1000 dollars for the candy. Who wants to eat one candy bar that costs that much? I don't think you would feel good, or honest, in destroying your body. Most people don't think in these terms but it's about time we do—by the time you retire, you may be so sickly that you cannot enjoy life.

One day I ate organic figs and felt great. I wondered what would happen if I ate three figs from the supermarket. So I did, and found that I developed sores in my mouth. Then I ate ten figs fresh from an unsprayed tree and had no problems.

My uncle grew up on a large peanut farm in the South. He told me, "I was down watching produce being shipped. I saw a man boxing the same fruit in the organic boxes as in the regular boxes, although he would take the smallest, worst-looking fruits for the organic boxes. I asked the man how he got away with this. He said, 'They don't know the difference. Besides, my chemicals are organic.'"

After listening to a lecture by Rachel Solomon at the Hippocrates South Institute in Lemon Grove, California, I asked about her experience with buying organic food. Rachel said, "I bought organic fruit and vegetables from a local farmer for five years. At the end of this time, I found out that the produce was not organic. The farmer had lied, charged double the price, and gave us the smallest, worst-looking food."

Because of abuses, there are now control groups to certify that the organic labeled foods are what they claim to be. The labeling and supervision of products is extremely important. The rules should be that everything that goes into and onto food must be told.

Labels must say:

| Waxed
| Radiated
| Acid/alkaline ratio of fruits and vegetables when picked
| Nutrients in the soil
| Nutrients in the plants
| Pesticides used—isolates
| If the nutrients feeding plants came from a whole form

In Philadelphia, you can walk into some Health Food Stores and buy beautiful organic groceries. They have everything you would need for optimum health. I always smile to myself as to how empty the aisles are. No one here fights for space. I know that, one day, this will change and will be like California. In San Diego, you constantly bump shoulders in trying to get at the organic food.

When people get more educated, we will see designer fruit and vegetables grown with "perfect soil," and "perfectly picked" labels. Our spendable income will go towards developing a longer, healthier life.

DEFINING TERMS

Organically Grown: Raised without synthetically compounded pesticides, herbicides, fungicides or fertilizers. Organically composted materials replenish soil humus content; mineral content is replenished by natural compounds such as bone meal, kelp and wood ash. Crops are not irradiated or treated with preservatives, hormones or other synthetic chemicals.

Certified Organic: Crops and soil are free of synthetic chemicals for one to three years depending on the state and certifying group. Inspections of farm and processing facilities verify organic methods, while soil testing is performed by an independent certifying group.

Transitional: A crop that has changed from synthetic chemicals to organic. The crop will be in a state of transition for three years. When all pesticide tests are lower than three years prior, the crop should be labeled "organic."

The FDA's pesticide monitoring report, *Residues in Food-1989*, reveals that almost 99 percent of the US grown products tested, and 96 percent of the imports, either showed no detectable pesticide residues or a level well below the legal limits permitted by the Federal Government.

I wonder about the legal limit of pesticides and nutrients because of my personal experience with organic and non-organic illustrates a big difference.

Bananas from the organic health food store are half the size of those from the supermarket. What do farmers do to make supermarket bananas twice the size of the organic? I don't know, although they are given a ripening gas. Organic bananas taste completely different; they are much sweeter and easier to digest. I can still taste chemicals even when I combine non-organic and organic bananas together. Organic celery is darker green than non-organic. I need only eat one piece at a sitting because the nutrients are so high. Although non-organic celery appears larger, I need to eat three sticks in one sitting to satisfy my appetite.

Organic apples are sweeter. I can definitely taste the chemicals on the non-organic apples. Organic oranges are picked at the right time for an acid/alkaline balance, making them more easily digestible. The color of organic oranges is an intense orange color, and taste three times sweeter than the non-organic.

In their book, *Live Food,* George and Doris Fathman write, "This is when we began to realize that almost all store food is junk food, whether packaged or not. It is raised on land that is dead from years of chemicals poured on to it. The result? Dead soil, dead food. And dead food doesn't support a live body. We learned, sadly, that one can slowly starve on three square meals a day when all you buy comes from the supermarket."

IRRADIATED FOODS

What is irradiated food? Did you know that our US Department of Energy (DoE) is spending millions of our tax money to build and test market irradiated food? Irradiated food is food treated with cesium-137 a highly radioactive material with a half-life of 30.2 years and a hazardous life span of 600 years. Corium-137 is defense waste and was one of the major radioactive materials emitted into the atmosphere by the Soviet Union's Chernobyl nuclear plant accident and is easily absorbed into our food chain. In October 1987, cesium-137 contaminated over 240 people in Goiania, Brazil. Several people died and many face an increased prospect of cancer and sterility. The accidental exposure occurred when cesium-137 was scavenged from an abandoned medical facility and ended up in the local junkyard.

Why would our government want to radiate our food?

"On May 2, 1990 the FDA issued a rule defining the use of irradiation calling it a safe and effective means to control a major source of food-borne bacteria in raw chicken, turkey, and other poultry.

"Since 1963, the FDA has passed rules permitting irradiation to curb insects in foods and microorganisms in spices, to control parasite contamination in pork, and to retard spoilage in fruits and vegetables.

"But when it comes to food irradiation the only danger is to the bacteria that contaminate the food. The process endangers their genetic material, so the organisms can no longer survive or multiply."[1]

---

[1] Dale Blumentahal, "Food Irradiation, Toxic to Bacteria, Safe for Humans," *FDA Consumer—November 1990*, III, pp. 11, 12, 13, 15, 32.

Don't you think if organisms cannot multiply in irradiated foods that this may suggest treated foods may be dangerous to the human body. My belief is foods must possess live energy in order for humans to benefit from them.

In the *FDA Consumer Magazine*, Nov. 1990 issue, the article on "Food Irradiation Toxic to Bacteria Safe for Humans" says, "Irradiation is used to control insects and bacteria on food. It is perfectly safe and harmless. We are now using it on all poultry and fish to prevent salmonella poisoning."

Irradiation may also be used on potatoes and herbs sold in the supermarkets. Consumers are supposed to see an irradiation FDA symbol of a "radura" flower. If you look for this label in a supermarket chances are you will never see it, because it seems the stores are not displaying it.

Mike, of Peoples Medical Society, says, "A new law has been established. If you're making apple pie and two of the five ingredients have been irradiated, there is no need for the 'radura' label." The pretty flowery label magically can disappear.

Common sense says if we are given 80 chest x-rays, this would damage us by taking away our life energy. Plants are the same way. The more they are heated by radiation the less life energy they have and the more likely we will become sick from eating it.

CHEMICALS IN THE HOME

People unknowingly accumulate toxins in their bodies due to constant exposure to chemicals in their homes and offices. The toxins can end up in their brain cells and liver and may cause a weakness throughout their bodies. Dr. Harold D. Buttram, a Pennsylvania MD and expert in Environmental Chemicals and Human Illness, offers many ways we can choose to live in a natural environment. He writes in his article, *Chemicals in the Home*, "Fundamentally, there are three classes of chemicals which may cause illness in the home. These are: formaldehyde, volatile hydrocarbons, and pesticides."

I will never forget my daughter at age one becoming sick one evening when her bronchial tubes became so irritated that she coughed continuously. After the second night of this, I became alarmed because her mucous had thickened and lay heavily in her chest. I immediately took her to the doctor. The pediatrician asked if I had put new carpeting in her bedroom. He said she had formaldehyde poisoning and suspected that it came from a new carpet since the pediatrician himself had gotten formaldehyde poisoning after staying in a hotel that had installed new carpeting. I said, yes I had installed a new carpet pad. So when we got home I took her out of her bedroom and put her in mine. Within three days she started to clear up. I removed the new carpet pad but not the carpet and put her back into her bedroom. She proceeded to get sick again; therefore I had to take the carpet outside and leave it in fresh air until it could release the poisons. After this my daughter was fine, although when she gets a cold she seems to have a slightly weakened bronchial system.

Dr. Buttram says, "Of all the potentially toxic chemicals in the home or work place, formaldehyde causes the greatest extent of harm to human health. Radiolabelled formaldehyde, because of its lipid solubility, is taken up in over five times higher concentration in the brain than in other tissues.

"Formaldehyde disrupts cellular membranes, causing increased cellular permeability. It is attracted to chromosomes, where it causes cross-linkages with RNA and DNA molecules. It has a snowballing effect in that formaldehyde sensitivity, once developed, tends to extend to other chemicals.

"Symptoms of formaldehyde toxicity may involve any organ system of the body, but they tend to be primarily cerebral. Inability to concentrate, headaches, fatigue, dizziness and poor coordination are among major symptoms. Other symptoms are skin, throat and eye irritation, respiratory disorders, allergies, and increased reactivity with continued exposure.

"Normal houses contain 0.03 parts per million (ppm) of formaldehyde in household air. Environmental agencies recommended less than 0.02 ppm. When urea foam formaldehyde insulation (UFFI) is used much higher levels are found, averaging 0.12 ppm. UFFI is now banned, but few people realize that formaldehyde levels in shopping malls, mobile homes, office buildings, and energy efficient homes today commonly exceed by far the 0.12 ppm levels found in homes with UFFI.

"Also, it is seldom realized that high levels of formaldehyde may persist for a number of years in a house containing formaldehyde treated woodwork furnishings, according to documented studies of formaldehyde in mobile and UFFI homes."

Formaldehyde is used in many commercial products, including permanent-pressed clothes, belts, leather products, wood paneling, plywood, particle boards, furniture sealants, carpets and products that have been glued. It is also used in rubber, metals, plastics, cosmetics, toiletries, medications, mattresses, latex paint, and adhesives. Major sources in the home come from glues used in plywood, particle boards, wall to wall carpets, and furniture sealants. Indoor combustion sources include invented gas stoves and kerosene heaters.

Dr. Buttram also has identified many pollutants and substances that contain them and some corrective measures as follows:

CARPETS, PLYWOOD, CABINETS, PARTICLE BOARD, AND PANELS: Largely because of their content of glues, cements, and adhesives, these fixtures exude or "outgas" such chemicals as phenols, acetone, toluene, xylene, benzene, polystyrene, ethanol, styrene, and formaldehyde. From a chemical standpoint (if one has a choice), plaster walls or untreated wood (free of formaldehyde) are best. Wall to wall carpets should be avoided; cotton throw rugs are best.

BEDDING: Foam rubber pillows and mattresses outgas harmful chemicals. Cotton mattresses may be laced with pesticides and fire retardants. Safe products are available.

FLOOR CLEANING MATERIALS IN COMMON USE: Phenol, formaldehyde, toluene, xylene, and methylene chloride.

METHYLENE CHLORIDE: Solvents in paints, varnish removers, aerosols, lacquers, hair sprays, and decaffeinated coffee.

STYRENE: Synthetic rubber, resins, soft plastics, coffee cups, meat trays in grocery stores.

PHENOLS: Disinfectants, soft plastics, television wires when overheated, cough medications, preservatives in many injectable medications.

XYLENE: Solvents, many commercial products, cleaning fluids, pesticides, dewaxers, glues.

METHANOL: Duplication fluids, copy machines, varnishes, dyes, paint thinners. Methanol is a metabolite of the common commercial sweetener, Nutrasweet. It is converted in the body into formate.

ETHYLENE GLYCOL: Paint solvents, anti-freeze, inks.

SMOKING: Probably the greatest single source of indoor air pollution. It is the source of 1,500 known chemicals, including aldehydes, aluminum, cadmium, benzopyrenes, formaldehydes, carbon monoxide, and outlawed pesticides.

GAS HEATERS WITH INADEQUATE VENTILATION: Sulfur dioxide, nitrous oxide, carbon monoxide, formaldehyde, other hydrocarbons.

TRICHLOROETHYLENE: Aerosol sprays, white-out(for typing corrections), solvents, dry cleaning.

CHLOROFORM: From heated chlorinated water, as when taking a hot shower.

MOTHBALLS: 100 percent parachlorobenzene.

DEODORANT SOAPS: Trichloroban, formaldehyde, phenols, ammonia.

POLYCHLORINATED BIPHENOLS (PCBs): These tend to persist in the environment. They are found in pump oils, hydraulic fluids, lubricating fluids, plastics on wires, carbonless paper, caulking, inks, paints, adhesives, flame retardants.

POLYBROMINATED BIPHENYLS (PBBS): Fire retardants.

VINYL CHLORIDE: Plastics, synthetic rubbers.

BENZENE: Solvents, cleaners, unleaded gasoline.

SOFT VINYL FLOOR TILE: Butanols, trichloroethylene, toluene, benzene, xylene, and phenols. Hard vinyl tile is relatively inert and safe.

12

SIGHT/ART

We don't normally think color is an indicator of the nutritional quality of food. But it is and we should try to get all colors of food into our diet each week..

Dr. Gabriel Cousens writes, "The color of food is key to the energy pattern of food and how its biomolecular nutrients will be bonded to specific cells and tissues in our bodies. The color of a food is its signature. As we become sensitive to nature's effort to communicate to us through her beautiful colors, we begin to develop a sensitivity to the particular food colors we are drawn to on a specific day as a key to what food energies and nutrients we need to balance our body. The Rainbow Diet is an acknowledgment of nature's effort to communicate with us."[1]

Try envisioning color of foods for your visual needs. Some examples of food colors are:

Yellow: apple, melon, grapefruit, banana, squash, pear, plum

Orange: apricot, cantaloupe, carrot, nectarine, orange, papaya, peach, sweet potato, tangerine

Red: apple, beet, cherry, grape, grapefruit, radish, raspberry, strawberry, tomato, watermelon

Purple: cabbage, turnip, grape

Blue: blueberry, cranberry, plum

Brown: Date, persimmon, pineapple, nuts, wheat

Green: apple, asparagus, broccoli, cucumber, grape, pea, pear, Romaine lettuce, wheat grass

White: artichoke, cabbage, cashew, cauliflower, chickpea, coconut, garlic, iceberg lettuce, lima bean, onion

---

[1] Gabriel Cousens, MD, *Spiritual Nutrition and the Rainbow Diet*, pp.19, 17, 74, 135, 136.

You might surmise that watermelon could be a good source of iron. Compare one 4 inch by 8 inch wedge of it to other foods. You can see that it truly is one of the best food source for iron.

Food	Iron Content
	(mg)
1 med orange	.72
1 apple	.39
1 cabbage	.80
1 cup of human milk	.08
1 grapefruit	1.14
1 4"x 8" wedge watermelon	4.63

Our government recommended daily allowance for iron is 15 mg for both adults and children. It would be easy to obtain this by eating watermelon.

Eyesight is very important to our health. Eyes allow a visual way to strengthen our immune system. People are now exploring Art Therapy, colored gems, crystals, metals and sunlight as means to improve their health.

Research has shown that one hour of sunlight exposure a day (without sunglasses) can stimulate our body function just as the sun does to a plant. When I become sluggish I sit in the sunlight for an hour and become revitalized.

"Color beamed into the aura of a living cell causes electrical reaction and transmutation to take place. Colour Therape (also known as Chromotherapy) is the art of using different colours to change or maintain vibrations to a frequency which will restore health and harmony to the human body and mind...Magenta is the color that combines infrared and ultraviolet and unblocks emotional problems by stimulating the correct vortex spin...If the body is to transmute the proper minerals, the colors have to be balanced 30 degrees apart in frequency. One just doesn't take any old red or blue. Color therapy is frequency! The numbers listed below the degrees are the Angstrom units of the colors. Angstrom is a unit used in measuring the length of light waves. An Angstrom unit is one-tenth of a millimicron. Note that green and magenta have the same Angstrom measurement. Both green and magenta are balanced midpoint between ultraviolet and infrared.

(Chemical elements)

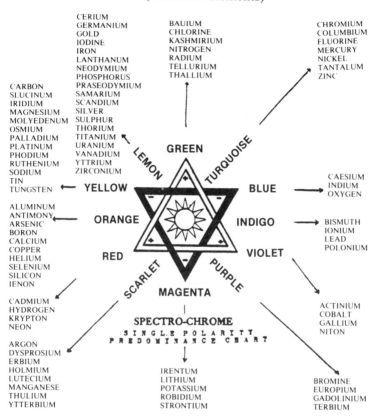

POSITIONS OF ILIUM, MASURIUM = UNDETERMINED.
RHENIUM = YELLOW. HAFNIUM, PROTOACTINIUM = LEMON

Chemical Elements By Single Color Polarity Predominance

From *Spectro-Chrome Metry Encyclopedia,* Dinshah, New Jersey, 1939.

"Optical wave lengths and color frequencies can initiate the transformation of a physical body. The chart shows how elements may be classified by their single color polarity. Red is shown to have four elements, the main one being hydrogen. Blue has only three elements, oxygen being the principal one. When hydrogen (red) and oxygen (blue) combine they make water. But before this chemical transformation can take place, there must first be an electrical stimulus. The two opposite polarity colors accomplish that. In the same way color beaming into a living cell causes the electrical reaction for a cell transformation.

"Example: A fever indicates that there is too much hydrogen in a person's body. If the wave length of oxygen, which is blue, is beamed onto the body, the oxygen will combine with the body's hydrogen and initiate the formation of water. This chemical reaction will release chemical energy and the person will break out into a sweat. This is called the process of transmutation. This process can only take place when the living energy field is present and in balance in the body."[1]

In *The Chemistry of Man* Bernard Jensen writes, "I began to do color experiments to find what effect color had on plant life. I created a red "green house" and saw how plants in their early stages grew twice as fast as they did in the regular greenhouse. Then I put plants in a blue "greenhouse" which caused them to be stunted. I felt that there was a story coming out in the use of colors. I wondered why someone hadn't been using colors in a therapeutic way.

"It might be difficult to see distinctions between a blade of grass and a geranium, yet there is a world of difference due to subtle dimensions beyond measure. The green color of the geranium contrasts to the green of the blade of grass, indicating the presence of more nitrogen, oxygen and calcium. The blade of grass contains more silicon, because it is likely to grow where the wind will blow on it, and the silicon will contribute to its resilient quality. Such subtleties in plants are transferred to us when we consume them."

Color guides us to the properties of plants. Magnesium, for example, is found in its highest concentration in yellow

[1] Dean Hardy, Mary Hardy, Marjorie Killick and Kenneth Killick, *Paramid Energy*, p. 104, has more information.

corn. Seasonal change, colors becoming brighter with summer and darker with winter, are reflected in our nutritional needs. I notice I crave completely different foods in the winter than in the summer. In winter my body needs more nuts, whereas in summer, with all the vitamin D coming from the sun, I have no interest in nuts.

Sunlight has a direct relationship with the retina of our eye. It is very important not to wear sunglasses while sun bathing because sunglasses block the nutrients from reaching our bodies. And we should never look directly into the sun because direct sunlight is too damaging for our eyes.

One simple way to experience color is through rocks. They can be small and easily placed any where in your house or worn on your body. In *Edgar Cayce On The Power Of Color, Stones, and Crystals*, Dan Campbell writes:

"Each color has its own vibratory pattern and its own special energy to offer you in bringing the miracle of metaphysical healing to yourself and loved ones. Colors, like snowflakes, are all different. Some offer you increased energy, while others bring you the gift of tranquillity. Through the use of your energized mind you can surround yourself with the energies of the color that offers you the quickest road to perfect health. Aided by your higher self you can also select clothing of colors which will be of greatest benefit to you in the area of metaphysical healing..."

In *Cunningham's Encyclopedia of Crystal, Gem & Metal Magic*, Scott Cunningham provides keys to the use of naturally occurring mineral colors:

Red: ruby, red jasper, red agate, rhodonite, red tourmaline, garnet. *"Symbolizes anger or other destructive emotions, birth, change, sex, passion, endings, energy confrontations."*

Pink: pink tourmaline, rose quartz, pink calcite, rhodcroste, kunzite. *"Symbolizes love, friendship, peace, joy, relationships, family interchange."*

Orange: carnelian, amber, citron, tiger's-eye coral. *"Symbolizes illumination, personal power, energy, growth."*

Yellow: yellow tourmaline, topaz, yellow fluorite. *"Symbolizes protection, communication, travel, exchange."*

Green: jade, peridot, olivine, aventruine, emerald, green tourmaline. *"Symbolizes, growth, money, grounding, health, fertility, business transaction."*
Blue: celestite, aquamarine, sodalite, blue quartz, blue tourmaline, turquoise, sapphire. *"Symbolizes peace, sleep, healing, purification, emotions, subconscious."*
Purple: sugllite, lepidolite, amethyst.
"Symbolizes spirituality, evolution, mysticism, expansion reincarnation."
White: diamond, quartz, white chalcedony, moonstone. *"Symbolizes God, peace, purity."*
Black: jet, obsidian, smoky quartz, black tourmaline, hemalite, hetconrite. *"Black stones are receptive, symbolic of self-control, of resilience and quiet power, absence of light."*

ART

Art is a mirror of our society and it can be a message to the viewer. Bruce M. Holly writes in "Psychology of Creativity," appearing in *Art Calendar Magazine*, that "Artists are individuals who have accepted the task of being conscious, and acting on their consciousness. By being willing, and able, to express emotions so that others can perceive and understand them, artists serve society by allowing us as an audience to learn about empathy without having to expose ourselves too directly to the raw emotions of real life. As the audience, our involvement with the thoughts and feelings contained in art is defined and limited, and we are not asked, usually, to expose our own discomfort with life.

"Art is a means of indirect experience for many, and is a catalyst for reliving and catharsis for some. As such, it demands courage and honesty from everyone involved, maker and viewer. By so doing, we learn not merely to understand, but to appreciate our lives, and ourselves."

It is now time for the artist to find the truth of our existence from not only a scientific or religious viewpoint, but from incorporating art, science and religion as one. Omraam Mikhael Aivanhov writes in *Creation: Artistic and Spiritual:* "Only art has the power, nowadays, to touch men profoundly and awaken them to the true life. This does not mean that no criticism can be made of the forms assumed by art today, on the contrary: in fact it would be true to say that it is very, very far from the ideal of art as the initiates understand it; an activity in which both true science and true religion are united. And yet, it is art that will save the world, an art that is conscious and enlightened by the truths of wisdom and love. In the future, artists will rank first in human society, for a true artist is priest, philosopher and scientist. Yes, for the function of an artist is to carry out on the physical plane that intelligence conceives as truth and the heart feels as good, in order to permit the world above, the world of the spirit, to descend and become incarnate in matter."

Artists are able to express themselves through a medium and reflect their inner thoughts. I, too, believe the only way we will help the world grow stronger is though the Artist.

Back to raw foods again, I noticed an incredible difference in my eyesight when changing my diet to raw. My world became alive in color—the reds, greens, blues, and yellows were brilliant. Never had I seen color like this before. My paintings started to become brighter than ever. In *Blatant Raw Foodist Propaganda!*, Joe Alexander writes,

"You see, as an artist, when I ate cooked foods I painted bleak, grotesque surrealist-type pictures with drab and dull, muddy colors; I was a creator of deserts in my art, but when I became a raw food eater, all of a sudden I began to paint instead, vibrantly alive pictures with lust abundance of healthy shapes and brilliantly beautiful colors, like the sort of lush jungle growth that Reich said was created by a strong concentration of healthy orgone energy in the atmosphere of an area."

My daughter, as well, draws and paints with brighter colors than I have ever seen a child use. Since the cooked foods leave more of a coating on the intestines, it creates a dull outlook on life. Scrub the inside with herbs and raw foods, and shine it up new! The art I create expresses the whole person with emphasis on the five senses—a thinking art that in some paintings can be felt, smelled or heard.

Why does a painting have to be square as if it is a window. The art of the future will completely break away from square art; shapes art will dominate the art world. Why does a painting consist of only one painting to express yourself? A painting can tell a story in which you could need 4, 6, or 8 paintings in a row to express your idea. Art does not need to express a gut feeling of negative emotion. Art can feel beautiful. Art can teach about life. Art can lift one's consciousness to a higher level!

The paintings on the following pages may be ordered in color numbered and signed prints, see the order form at the back of this book.

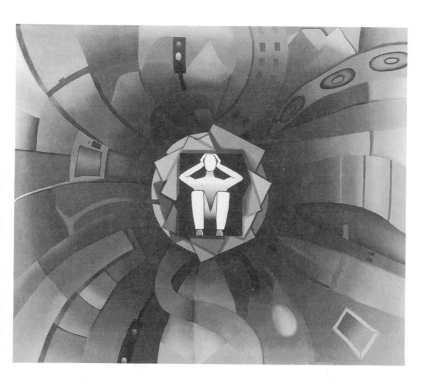

Listen From Within   38" x 40"   Oil on canvas

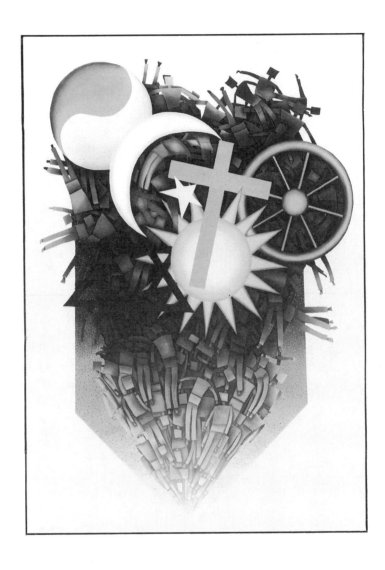

We All Come From One 73" x 40" Oil on canvas

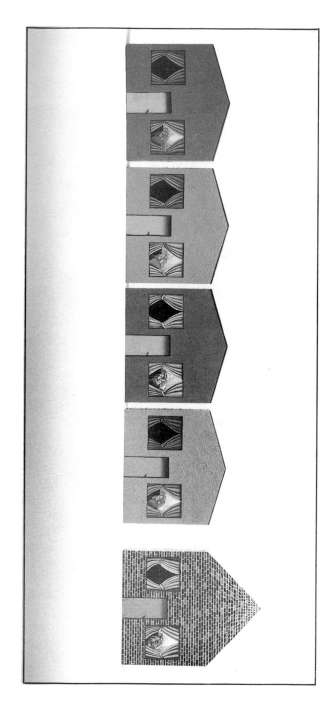

Little Boxes   10" x 60"   Oil on wood
Dinners depicting fish, pig, cow, chicken and vegetarian meals.

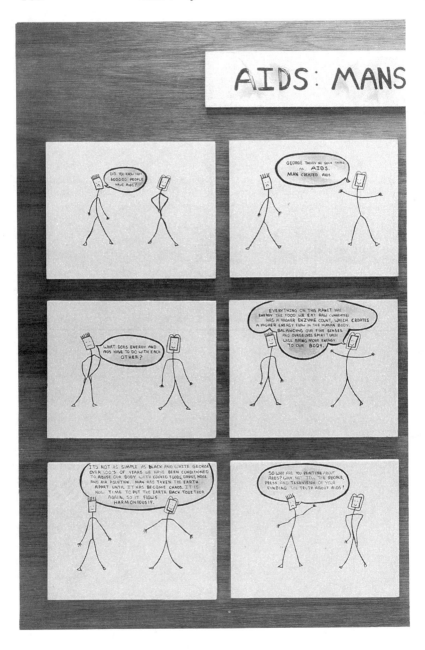

Aids: Man's Teacher

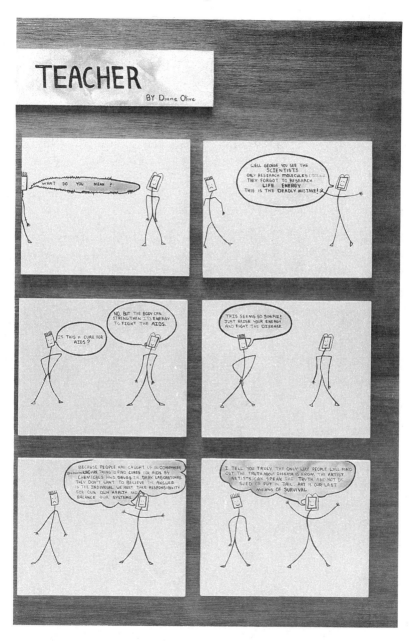

38" x 51"

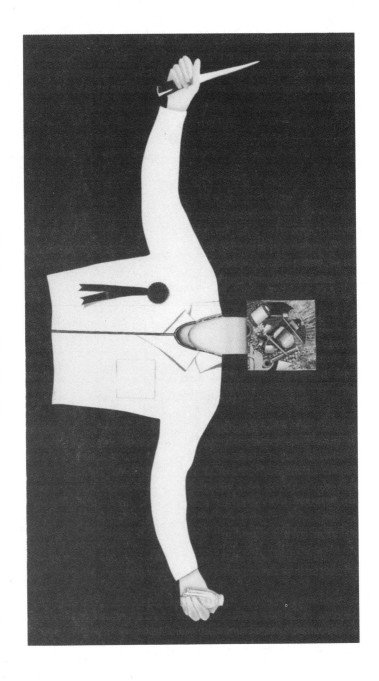

The Holy Men   30" x 65"   Oil on wood

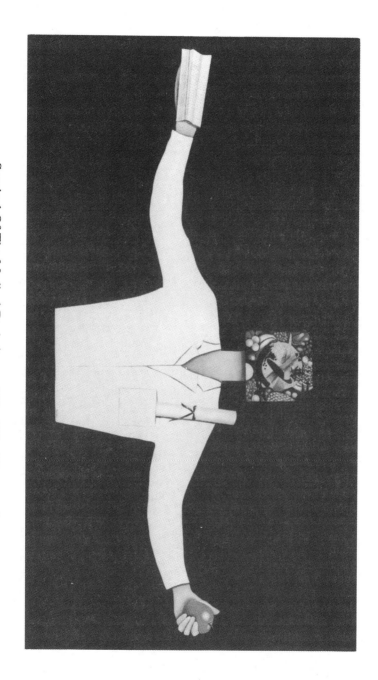

Survival Of The Medical Dark Ages   30" x 65"   Oil on wood

Spin To Become One   73" x 40"   Oil on canvas

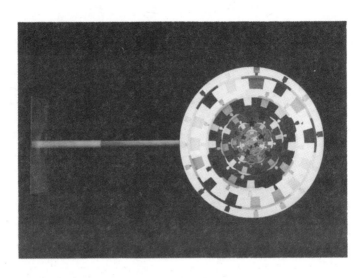

Same Painting Spinning

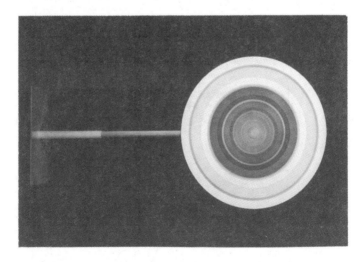

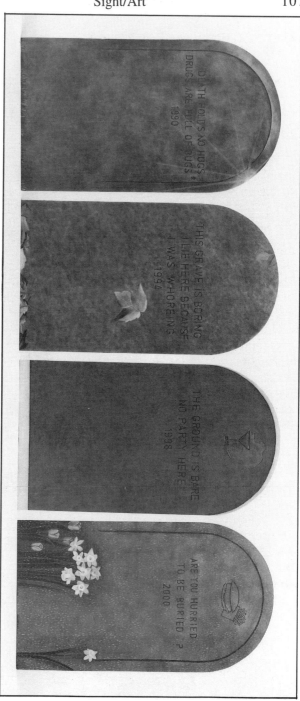

Death In The Four Seasons   27" x 63"   Oil on wood

13

SMELLS

I was walking up a hospital staircase when I took in a deep breath and smelled the odor of pure cement. Abruptly, there came over me a rush of emotion and memory. The smell reminded me of myself, as a child, walking up my grandmother's steps to her apartment. I used to walk up and down the enclosed staircase because I enjoyed the odor of the cement.

Odors reach into all of our emotional life, drawing from the deepest recesses in our minds. Odors suggest and stimulate associations, evoke, frighten, and arouse us, but seem to be below conscious thought. Most unpleasant smells warn of danger. Odors help bond mother and baby. Animals, to protect themselves from being poisoned, will rarely touch any food that smells like the one that made them ill.

In *National Geographic*, September 1986, Boyd Gibbons writes, "The sense of smell is at the heart of remembering and emotion. It's a matter of anatomy. Odors are volatile molecules. They float in the air. When you sniff, they rush through your nostrils, over spongy tissue that warms and humidifies the air, and up two narrow chambers where, just beneath the brain and behind the bridge of the nose, they land on a pair of mucus-bathed patches of skin the size of collar buttons. Here, in a process that's still a mystery, the molecules bind to receptors on tiny hair-like cilia at the ends of the olfactory nerves, or neurons, which fire the message to the brain."

Dr. Pasquale Graladei, a neurologist at Florida State University in Tallahassee, said, "If you damage a nerve cell of your brain, you will never regain it. Lose the cells of your spinal cord, you have paralysis. Blow the neurons in your retina or your ear, and you cannot repair the damage. Since olfactory nerve cells can be replaced, the sense of smell has to be very important. Nature doesn't ever do anything for fun.

"Some years ago my mother, a former, nurse, suspected that a neighbor might have stomach cancer when she detected the familiar odor of fermentation on his breath. In the days before high-tech medicine, physicians depended on all their senses, including their noses, to diagnose illness. An eminent diagnostician might arrive on a hospital ward, sniff, and announce that a case of typhoid fever must be in. Typhoid smelled like baking bread. German measles smelled like plucked feathers, scrofula like stale beer, yellow fever like a butcher shop. A surgeon on rounds will ordinarily smell the patient's bandage for infection by pseudomonas bacteria. It has the musty odor of a wine cellar."

The laboratory has drawn physicians away from their senses and their patients.

Egyptians four thousand five hundred years ago thought that bad odors caused disease, and pleasant ones chased disease away. Some Romans slept on pillows stuffed with saffron in an attempt to avoid the feared Black Death epidemic. In nineteenth century Europe, physicians made their rounds carrying aromatics to ward off the plague and its stench.

Perhaps humankind must completely rule out the manufacture of synthetic odors. We don't need to compete with nature. Regenerating and maintaining health through naturally occurring perfumes is the only way to have a lasting positive effect.

Aromatics are different essences extracted from flowers, plants, and animals. Some smell good, others bad. They were the backbone of Egyptian medicine. Before synthetic perfumes doctors were able to get patients to sleep without harmful effects, just by using natural aromatic from plants such as: Italian citrus, orange blossom, rose, geranium, and lavender. They were able to relax patients by putting rose aromas into their bath water. It is obvious that smell therapy, in the future, will be a major way to achieve healing.

Aroma therapy is the art and science of using the essential oils of flowers and plants for beautifying and healing purposes. Aroma therapy is a holistic approach to well-being which promotes relaxation and rejuvenates or stimulates body, mind and spirit.

Lilaila O. Afrika writes in *African Holistic Health,* about the different uses (not for internal use) of oil/incense:

Oil/incense	Uses
myrrh	nasal congestion, energy
olibanum/frankincense	aids birth muscles, vasoconstrictor, nervous system
jasmine/calamus root	blood purifier, kidney tonic, mineral stabilizer
pine/burnt pine cones	respiration system, digestive organ cleanser, energy, regulator,rejuvenator
lavender/styrax	cleanser of glands and skin, curative
oakmoss/cedar	blood purifier, digestion, nerves
rose/sandalwood	cleanser, nerves, pituitary gland

14

SOUNDS/HEARING

"Awareness is a form, and a form or action is made up of light, and light is sound, and sound-energy is music. Therefore, only through fine attunement with Earth-awareness, Earth music can we reach our highest goodness." (Joseph Rael in *Spiritual Ecology*)

There are now instruments with sounds that can be beamed into the body's energy points to diagnose a disease. The sounds of the instrument will come out unclear if there is something wrong. Technology has also brought us instruments where beneficial sounds are beamed into the organ to heal it.

The effect of music and sound on the human being is very important to Health. Researchers are now, discovering how certain kinds of music and 'sound can contribute to stress tension' headache, nausea, loss or disturbed sleep, poor digestion irritability, lack of concentration, high blood pressure, and hyperactivity. Some sounds are found to be disturbing to the body and some sounds are therapeutic.

There are natural laws in the universe based on vibration of rhythm or oscillation. For example experiments have been done on clocks with pendulums, by placing all clocks in the same room the pendulums will naturally follow order and become in sync with each other. We are visibly aware of the universal law when we observe the pendulums swinging in the exact pattern together. Duplication of this pendulum experiment can be done with females. In many cases when women live together they start to experience their female cycles synchronized and they start their menstruation on the same day.

Every cell in the body has vibratory properties and is a sound receptor. The body vibrates at a certain rate of 7.8 to

8.0 cycles per second when relaxed. When we meditate or pray it is in a 8.0 cycles per second. The earth vibrates at the same fundamental frequency. When two or more thing vibrates together it is called entrainment. Entrainment must be understood to understand how the body functions to sound. The body resonates automatically to all incoming vibrating forces. When humans vibrate and harmonize together they have entrainment with each other. This entrainment can come from outside sounds that are lifting to our consciousness or lower our mental awareness.

Our hearts beat in rhythm of three. Our well being can be disrupted by Rap music or heavy Rock and Roll which are in a beat of two.

There are many sounds that are not even heard such as electrical ones which can change our bodies flow. Passing by a nuclear power plant or electrical wiring can alter our vibrational pattern, bringing us out of tune. In contrast, we must be aware of beautiful sounds that can vibrate and massage the tissues and cells which strengthen our immune system. There are patterns and rhythms everywhere we look. In the start of life we hear our mothers heart beat, then we hear our first breath in and out. Leisure music relaxes us while an up-tempo beat stimulates us.

"Experience tells us that some sounds *put* us to sleep (lullabies) and some keep us awake (traffic) some calm us (surf on the beach) and some make us dance all night *(rhythm)*. A hard driving beat practically forces us to tap our feet. The screech of chalk on a black board makes us scream and contract in discomfort. We are constantly bathed by sound." (Don Campbell in *Music Physician*)

I was told a true story of monks who chanted different sounds together every day. When a new younger monk came to the convent he decided to put a stop to this ancient singing. Soon after this the monks developed depression and illness. So they returned to their chanting and were once again fine.

Together with the wave lengths of color, sound vibration can transmute substances from one frequency to another.

Some sounds can vibrate our bodies to a more peaceful balance. I use the "om"" sound to relax and calm my mind. It takes me two minutes to "om" the body to a state of relaxation.

It is quite logical to realize that different notes of music vibrate different parts of the body. We can realize this by making different sounds—aw, ba, ma, la—remembering that our bodies beat at a particular rhythm in conjunction with the heartbeat. Beethoven figured out the rhythm of the human body and produced music to enhance this beat. Birds, the ocean, and some New Age music produce good sounds to stimulate the human body's natural rhythms.

HAVING RHYTHM WITH MOTHER EARTH

Our arms move in Rhythm.
We breathe in Rhythm.
Our hearts beat in Rhythm.
The body as a cycle Rhythm (for menstruation and ovulation)
Our bodies have a cleansing and rebuilding Rhythm.
A pentagon has Rhythm.
The sun has a cycle Rhythm.
A plant flowers in Mother Earth to a Rhythm.
Birds fly south in Rhythm.
We make music in Rhythm.
The planet, and everything on it,
functions together in Rhythm.

Lilaila O. Afrika writes in *African Holistic Health*: "Music sounds are another form of energy. They enter the human body by way of the skin, eyes, ears, and foods. The music sounds enter the body and stimulate the organs and have a healing effect. The notes can be sung, played on a musical instrument or heard as forms of healing."

THE EFFECT OF MUSICAL NOTES

D: For digestion and assimilation, diseases involving the lungs and the respiratory system.
G: Stimulates tranquillity and peace, eliminate infections.
C: Blood disease.
E: Purification, assists in healing diabetes, intestinal and bowel diseases.
B: Nervous systems, eye and brain injuries, and insomnia.
F: The nervous system, circulatory system and heart.
A: Diseases of eye, ear, nose, dental, and emotional disorders.

One day, there will be a major recognized practice of "vibration therapy." Scientists will realize that we are a vibrating electrical energy mass that can be balanced with beneficial sounds. At that time, probably all senses will be used together to form a complete therapy program.

15

TOUCH/EXERCISE

The history of massage can be traced as far back as 3,000 BC. Chinese, Indians, Egyptians, Persians, Japanese, Romans and Greeks believed firmly in the benefits of massage which were highly recommended as a means of helping the body to heal itself.

"Massage is also a gift because you are giving your time to someone. You could just as easily choose to pursue a favorite pastime like playing tennis or watching television. Instead, you have chosen to spend a certain amount of your time giving of yourself to someone special or someone in need.

"It is a known fact that massage improves circulation of the blood and lymph, and that most conditions will improve if the circulation of these two vital fluids is encouraged."[1]

"Not only do abnormally tight, tense muscles operate ineffectively, but they impede proper circulation as well. When the circulation is impaired, fresh blood is unable to reach and nourish the tissues, and waste products collect. This causes a decreased exchange of fluids within the tissues, leading to fatigue and a general imbalance within our body systems.

"Massage acts as a mechanical cleanser as it increases the interchange of tissue. Fluids emptied into the blood capillary and lymphatic network, removing the products of fatigue and inflammation. By doing this, massage indirectly increases the tone of the muscles being treated by passively increasing the contracting power of the muscles.

---

[1] Ouida West, MTH, *The Magic of Massage*, p.13

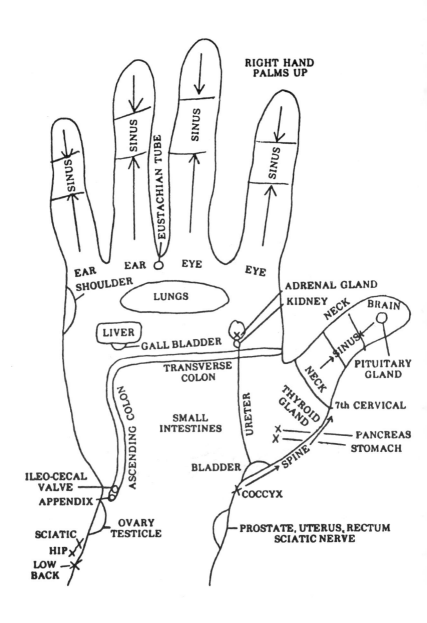

RIGHT HAND
PALMS UP

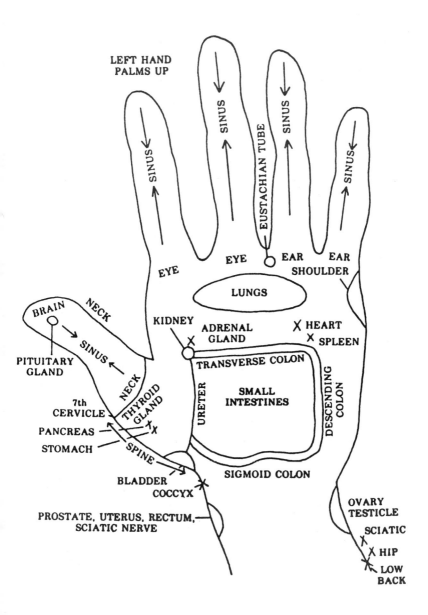

RIGHT

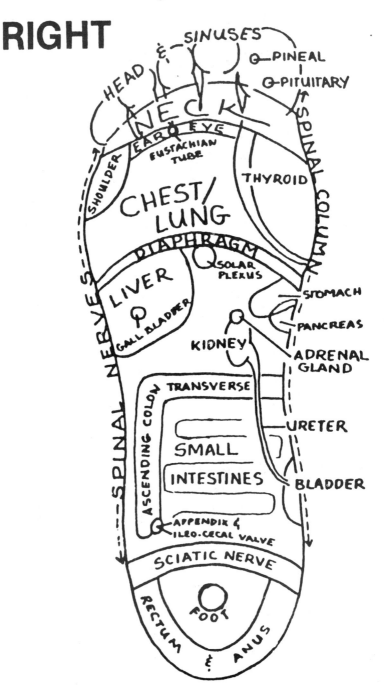

LEFT

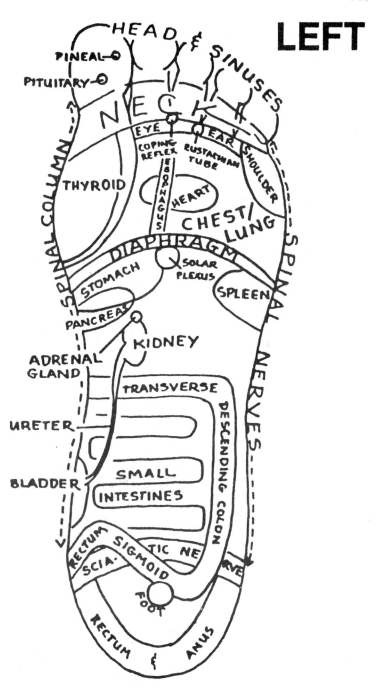

While bringing about a deep sense of relaxation, massage also improves circulation, helps maintain fluid balance, and relieves excess tension. Self massage is a personal way to help maintain your own well-being."[1]

If these energy points become blocked or stagnated, this will create imbalance and cause illness.

In *Immune System Activation*, John Selby writes about the importance of our hands touching our own bodies for healing. "As you relax, focus on your hands again and say the word 'healing' to yourself a couple of times. Just see how this word resonates in your system. Notice particularly if you do feel healing energy in your hands at this point. If not, fine, But if there is some energy available, you can breathe without effort, and let your hands move on their own, and go anywhere on your body that they want to, wherever healing energy and attention is needed at the moment, and say 'healing' when you want to, to enhance the process."[2]

Note: All our system's neural energies circulate through the feet and the hands. This is why the New Age doctors are finding medical problems by examining feet. Doctors now can press their fingers on the bottom of a foot to find and stimulate an organ. I was tested on all spots of my foot. They found the liver-gall bladder to be painful and it was, in reality, my problem. One year later, when I was much healthier and was retested, I had no more pain in the palm of my hand nor the bottom of my feet. Chinese doctors are quite familiar with these charts and have been practicing for thousands of years with this diagnosis.

"You can examine your own feet in the same way. As soon as you find a tender spot, press firmly with your thumb, while holding the breath, until the pain goes away. In this way, you will be giving yourself a healing treatment. Once you have examined and treated your own feet, relax your body as you have been instructed, and begin to send healing thoughts to the organ or organs that have been affected."[3]

---

[1] Monika Struna with Connie Church, *Self-Massage*, pp. 12-14.

[2] John Selby with Manfred Von Luhmann, MD, *Immune-System Activation*, p. 6.

[3] Ibid.

EXERCISE

WALKING

Walking exercises more muscles than running and probably is a better form of exercise for most people because this activity induces a very gentle massage of the bottom of the exerciser's foot. Foot nerves connect to all body functions; therefore, stimulation of the feet causes stimulation of all body functions.

"Walking briskly gets your heart pumping, your lungs working, and just about all the muscles and joints of your body exercised. It gives the same benefit as jogging and causes less wear and tear on the body. You'll find very few walkers in the waiting rooms of the podiatrists and orthopedists. At sixty or even seventy you can still walk with vigor.

"Research has shown that walking begun early in life slows the aging process.

"Mainly you want to remember not to put all your weight down hard on your heel. The outer part of the heel should hit the ground first and you roll along the outside of the foot and step off the ball of the foot, pushing with your toes."[1]

YOGA

I find Yoga to be the best form of stretching. Yogic exercise can help your body relax and feel better for the demands placed upon it. And a well trained body helps to train the mind. Yoga increases circulation and keeps arteries elastic, strengthens endocrine and cleanses the lymph system.

Yoga stresses the importance of flexibility of the spine in creating good health whereas aerobics works muscles, pounding them to hardness. Increased flexibility allows blood to flow unimpeded throughout a person's body and thereby boost blood supply to our tissues.

I noticed my posture becoming more aligned after I did the yoga exercises. One major benefit was to my back. It felt better than it had previously from all the other exercises (low impact and normal aerobics, stair climbing, stretching, etc.) I had tried.

[1] Jack Solfanoff, DA, *Natural Healing*, pp. 86-87.

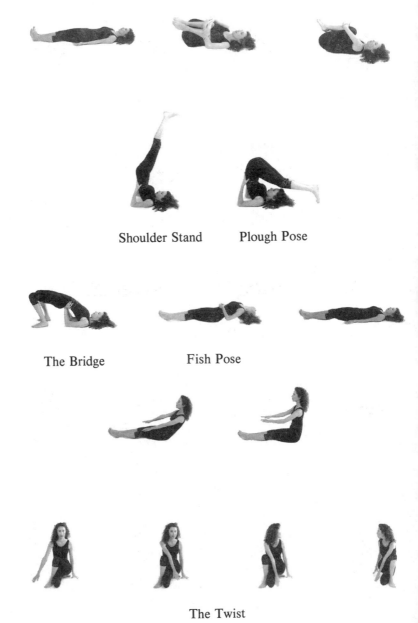

Shoulder Stand Plough Pose

The Bridge Fish Pose

The Twist

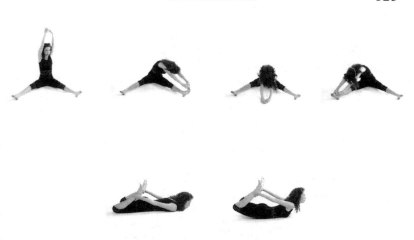

The Bow (Rocking back and forth)

The Cobra

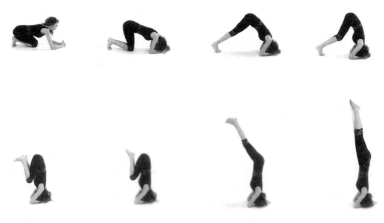

Going into a Headstand

It appears that Yoga can produce increased mental focus and deep relaxation in a person by a combination of stretching, deep breathing, and relaxation.

The preceding yoga exercises are the ones I found to be beneficial.

TAI CHI:
THE GREAT CIRCLE EXERCISE FORM

Many people I know do not seem to need the stimulations produced by active sports such as running, racquetball, tennis, etc. They feel they have found the ultimate exercise, Tai Chi. They claim this gentle exercise strengthens every function of the body even including our bones. Perhaps this will be the exercise of the future. But what is it?

"The Great Circle is a long, single routine consisting of portions of segments, some of which are repeated during the routine.

"All of the movements of Tai Chi are natural to the human body and enhance the normal functions of the human body.

"The movements of Tai Chi involve the whole body, from head to feet. Coordination is enhanced through the rhythmic, flowing style of the routine; balance and body gestures are improved."

Because there is no competition involved, Tai Chi promotes a relaxed mental attitude which transfers to relax the body. Coordination of eye-limb activity involves a degree of mental concentration which is stimulating and relaxing."[1]

REBOUNDING

A rebounder is a small round springy platform on legs that closely resembles a trampoline. A person exercises on it by standing in its middle and then bouncing up and down.

On it, if you choose, you can dance, body build with weights, or jog. People also may find that use of a rebounder will improve their coordination. Above all it can provide a safe low impact method for creating aerobic benefits and a cleansing of lymphatic systems.

---

[1] Bruce Teghers, *Kung Fu & Tai Chi: Chinese Karate and Clasical Exercises* (Thor Publishing Co., Ventura, CA), pp.87-88.

16

TASTE

Once in Hawaii I ordered a Pina Colada cocktail without alcohol. Almost immediately after placing the order, I had an urge to examine the ingredient labels of the coconut and pina banana mix bottles used to make the drink. "What chemicals are you putting into our drinks?" I wanted to ask, but I was afraid to because I knew the answer would be disturbing. I knew I would confirm it was dead food that had been sitting around in a bottle for six months or more. Even though the drink was tasty, the bartender could have created a tastier and healthier drink if he had known about live enzymes. I'm sure he would rather make a drink using fresh fruit which would be life-enhancing instead of life-taking.

Dates taste dark and rich to me whereas oranges taste juicy. Nature has made so many different tasting foods for us (carrots, celery, apples, bananas, etc.). We are so fortunate that we can eat from such a wide choice of foods.

We don't have to eat people-made food that causes disease. Basically, I put food into two categories:

Foods Straight From the Earth		People Manipulated Foods (Heated, Processed)	
Apples	Fruit	Cereal	Enriched
Corn	Grains	Boxed	Heated
Almonds	Nuts	Canned	Processed
Pumpkin	Seeds	Frozen	Preserved
Lettuce	Vegetables	Cured	

When you get past people-made food, you can taste the richness of Earth's clean foods. I never liked vegetables until I started eating herb foods. I believe the herb foods supplied nutrients I was lacking to clean up my palate. Now fresh foods taste wonderful and heated, processed foods taste lifeless.

There are fantastic dishes you can make with herbs— casseroles, creamy soups, sandwiches, tacos, dips, etc., all with delicious raw foods.

My best recipes can be found in Appendix 1.

17

MIND

Doctor's know that a patient with a good self-image and a positive outlook will survive a life-threatening disease more easily than the patient who is fearful, resigned, or grieving. They also know that the mind is powerful enough to create illness. Health, then, depends on our thoughts, i.e., whether they are positive or negative.

When I first heard this idea I was angry. I didn't want to believe that my illness might be caused by negative thoughts. I was aware that the body's tendency was to reveal illness where it is weak. Although illness appears to be inherited, it may be that we inherit weakness not disease. Still, we are responsible to strengthen our weaknesses. So I decided to look deeper into the possibility that our mind could really cause illness.

I found proof of this concept in an audio tape of W. Brugh Joy's book, *Personal and Collective Healing*. Dr. Joy, MD, reported very interesting research on people who had multiple personalities. He found that people with these kinds of disorders can have different diagnosed diseases for each of their personalities. For example, one person's illness could change from diabetes to allergies to skin rashes as their personality changed. I now realized that different diseases could be linked with the various personalities. In her books, Louise Hays goes through every disease and describes a personality that promotes the illness. For instance she writes, "I believe that we contribute to every illness in our body. The body, as with everything else in life, is a mirror of our inner thoughts and beliefs. Our body is always talking to us, if we will only take the time to listen. Every cell within our bodies responds to every single thought we think...When we discover what the mental pattern is behind an illness, we have a chance to change the pattern and, therefore, the dis-ease. Most people do not want to be sick on a conscious level, yet every dis-ease that we have is a teacher. Illness is the body's way of telling us that there is a false idea in our consciousness. Something that we are believing, saying, doing, or thinking is not for our highest good. I always picture the body tugging at us saying, please-pay attention!...We had both noticed, among innumerable clients and patients who were ill, a strong tendency to spend most of the time either thinking about the future or lost in the past reflections. Very little actual time was spent focused on the present moment. Thus very little conscious attention was being focused on the person's body right here, right now...But in basic biological time, it is only right here, right now within every ongoing moment, that the body actually heals itself. So a basic rule for encouraging immune system activation is this: Hold your attention focused here in the present moment."

When trying to create a positive life, a good way to start is to write down your visions, gifts, loved ones, and belief system. Then make a lists of negatives in your life. Examine the list to see if it is balanced or unbalanced in a direction that is causing you problems. If so, then make adjustments to bring your life back into balance. The following is an example.

Negative	Positive
School	Art
Cooked foods	Family
Pollution	Raw food
Sickness	God
Job	

When my school load was too negative, I switched schools instead of dropping out. A good idea is to work on the negatives one by one, so that they don't become overwhelming. Once you have changed a negative into a positive, learn the lesson from it and go on with your life. Don't dwell on the past, help be a creator.

I know when I was very sick and emotional problems arrived, I could not deal with them. For example, my mother-in-law would tell me I was too slow with my housework, not understanding I was to ill to do it. I could not handle criticism and any at all would make me sicker. Our minds and bodies are very affected by emotions and negative emotions can definitely make things worse. One of the healthiest things I did to get better was stay away from things that made me feel stressed.

Organized living is very important to me. Keeping my house neat and tidy contributes to me functioning better. I found, also, that taking one day each week for a day of rest and partial fasting was very important. Think about goal setting. No matter how staggering your goals might be you can always break them up into small pieces of time fragments such as: one hour of each day for painting, one hour for writing, two hours each morning for cleaning and one hour with my daughter for quality time. Setting goals and then arranging my life to reach these goals proved to be a major stepping stone in my life.

"Diet influences the state of mind, and the state of mind influences the diet choice....Consciously or unconsciously, people tend to choose the diet that reinforces and is reflective of their own mental and spiritual state of awareness."[1]

"We used to think allergies were causes for stuffed-up, runny noses and red eyes but new medical fields are showing people's mental functioning can be disrupted by the foods we eat and the pollutants they breathe. (Some food/environmental caused) Symptoms include acute and chronic depression, tension-fatigue syndrome, minimal brain dysfunction, restlessness, anxiety, insomnia, hyperactivity, inappropriate behavior outburst, fear, panic, unreal feelings, personality changes, schizophrenia, psychosis, hallucinations, and inability to concentrate."[2]

Scientists are now finding that a diet of cooked foods can cause brains to decrease in size. Scientist Edward Howell found brains of wild meadow mice are twice as heavy as those of tame laboratory mice. "When rats are given a 'factory' diet, body weight goes up and brain weight goes down. I have reached this conclusion by assessing more than 50 submitted in the scientific periodical literature over a number of years."[3]

---

[1] Gabriel Cousens, MD, *Spiritual Nutrition and the Rainbow Diet*, pp.19, 17, 74, 135, 136.

[2] Mandell, Marshall and Scanlon, Lynne Waller, *5-Day Allergy Relief System*.

[3] Dr. Edward Howell, *Enzyme Nutrition*.

Food can change our attitude. It can make us weak, strong, positive, negative. It can make our minds sharp and clear or foggy and spacy. I say this because I know when I've gone too far off my diet, or cheated too much on man-made foods, my mind becomes fuzzy and out of focus. Whereas with a complete raw diet, I have no such problem. My mind clicks in to process information and find correct words and answers.

In Napoleon Hill's *Laws of Success*, one of the greatest books ever written about achieving success, the author sets out certain principles to follow. Here are some of the chapter headings he uses.

1. Power—what it is and how to create and use it.
2. Cooperation—the psychology of cooperative effort and how to use it constructively.
3. The Master mind—how it is created through harmony of purpose and effort, between two or more people.
6. Imagination—how to stimulate it so that it will create practical plans and new ideas.
7. Telepathy—how thought passes from one mind to another through the other. Every brain is both a broadcasting and receiving station for thought.
10. Air and ether— how they carry vibrations.
18. How to analyze yourself.
22. Some reasons why people fail.
24. Why some people antagonize others without knowing it.
28. Chemistry of the mind— how it will make or destroy you.
30. The mind becomes devitalized— how to "recharge" it.
31. The value and meaning of harmony in all cooperative effort.
33. This is the age of mergers and highly organized co-operative effort.
36. Every human possesses at least two distinct personalities—one destructive and one constructive.
37. Education is generally misunderstood to mean instruction or memorization of rules. It should mean development from within, of our human mind through unfolding and use.
38. Two methods of gathering knowledge—personal experience and assimilation of knowledge gained by others

These Golden Rules should be taught in the lower school system. We learn so much data in school, but not enough practical knowledge that is the essential for humans to get along in life!

18

MENSTRUAL PERIOD

This information could be the most exciting breakthrough for women. I believe diet and menstruation are connected. The diet of raw foods (fruits, vegetables, nuts, seeds, sprouts and herbs) and staying within a similar protein content as human mother's milk can lower the days of the blood menstruation, cramping, and/or stop them altogether.

Why do our bodies bleed slowly each month? Could it be that we eat a diet too high in protein. This may cause a toxic build-up within us which we discharge once a month via our menstrual periods. I found that women do not have to have blood flows to ovulate and they can become pregnant.

1. What is the physiology of menstruation?
2. Is it a necessary accompaniment to ovulation?
3. Why do not all females the world over menstruate?
4. Why do healthy women not menstruate and the sickly menstruate at length?
5. Is menstruation functionless? If not, what is its function?

Lets take a close look at the menstrual cycle, and how we have thought it is formed.

"The menstrual cycle is governed by hormones produced by the pituitary glands and the ovaries. Estrogen and progesterone are the substances that the ovaries naturally manufacture under the direction of the master gland, the pituitary. With ordinary amounts of these hormones in the bloodstream, the pituitary gland signals the ovaries to release an ovum every month at the midpoint between the menstrual periods. When hormone levels are a little higher, as in pregnancy, the pituitary does not direct ovulation."[1]

What people are saying now is that there is no normal need for the release of blood every 28 days.

"Ovulation, in the healthy woman, occurs without menstruation. Menstruation occurring coincident with ovulation is not normal. Weak muscles in the abdominal area contribute to the hemorrhage condition that the menstruating woman experiences monthly. After the woman ovulates, there is a thickening of the mucous membrane lining the uterus in preparation for conception. In the healthy woman the mucous lining is passed out as a very slight mucous discharge when conception does not occur. The many fine capillaries diminish in number until preparation is again made for conception after normal ovulation. Due to a weakness of the capillary walls and excessive inflammation, the toxic woman experiences a hemorrhage of the uterus, a pathological condition, which, because of its near universality, she mistakes as part of the normal function of ovulation."[2]

The female body will stop menstrual blood flow for two reasons: She is too toxic or she is very healthy.

There are many cases where menstrual flow has stopped due to a highly toxic diet. The body is weakened to a point where it loses its ability to carry out the monthly cleansing process. As toxins continue to build up, unless there is a change in life style, the female will develop some chronic disorders.

When I changed my diet to more fruits and vegetables, I began to get healthier. My blood flow only lasted one day, gradually disappearing to become a light creamy colored discharge lasting one day with no cramping; however, the blood flow would come back if I ate "junk food". It must be that menstruation is a removal of toxic waste, a cleansing process.

"When toxic blood seeks an outlet through the womb via the menstrual function, the resulting inflammation and irritation to the delicate mucous membrane throws the organ

[1] Victoras Kulvinskas, MS, *Survival Into the 21st Century*, pp. 173, 118.

[2] Wendy Harris and Nadine Forrest McDonald, *Is Menstruation Necessary?* pp. 22, 29.

into spasms which are registered as pain or cramps. If the toxin is milder or more dilute, the patient simply feels heavy or congested in her pelvis. Once the flow has started, nature pours out as much toxic material from the blood as possible. This inflames the deeper layers of the womb. What should be a normal flow develops into a hemorrhage, some times lasting for days and reducing the patient to a state of anemia. The womb, weakened after such chemical poisoning, is easy prey to harmful bacteria" writes Dr. Bielar in the book *Natural Way to Sexual Health*. That is, when you lose blood you lose nutrients.

"Among the nutrients lost are lecithin, calcium phosphate, sodium chloride, alkaline lactates, sodium bicarbonate, potassium chloride, cholesterol, albumin, mucin, vitamins A and E, amino acids."[1]

"The discharge preceding menstruation (usually mucus) and is rich in the iodine, lecithin, and calcium elements. At this time women may experience depression, become apathetic and lethargic, and find themselves easily upset, and angry or crying. Women commit more suicides at this time than any other in their lives."[2]

"In the menstrual blood there is six times the number of sex hormones concentrated than in blood in general circulation. This periodic loss of sex hormones in a period of thirty to forty years of menstruation brings on the menopause, effecting loss of youth."[3]

Twenty percent of women who reach age thirty-five have pathological growths in the uterus. Forty percent of women who reach the age of forty have myomas (tumor of the muscle tissue). Myomas only happens when we have inflammation and thickening of the uterine mucous membrane or lining from blood flow. This is indicated by the fact that myomas never develop before the onset of menstruation or after menopause.

When I recall the excitement of starting my blood flow at the age of sixteen, I realize I was one of the last of my friends to be initiated into womanhood by this horrible pain and

[1] Ibid.

[2] Ibid.

[3] Survival Into the 21st Century, by Victoras Kulvinskas, M.S. pp. 118, 173.

smelly blood. Still, I was so excited to be like the rest, I never thought there was anything wrong with bleeding.

I would wake up at 2 o'clock in the morning with cramps. I couldn't sleep, so I would pace the floor back and forth, finally give in to Tylenol.

As I became sicker, my menstrual periods became longer. Instead of just one day of horrible pain, feeling like my stomach was being hit repeatedly with a bat, the pain persisted for four days straight and the bleeding continued for seven or more days.

Women who follow a diet closest to the nutrients of human mothers' milk cease heavy flow or decrease the amount of days for the flow.

Mrs. Pearl Briggs had many illnesses and was dying. Her husband, who desperately tried to help her, stumbled onto American Natural Hygiene (whole raw foods, herbs, fasting, vegetarian lifestyle). He then started applying these natural laws to his wife. Pearl said "I started feeling really good on this diet and all my health problems vanished. Also, my once a month blood flow disappeared. I was concerned, but had read that when the body works properly this will lighten and then disappear to a discharge more like a light cream. I went to my medical doctor who said I would never get pregnant without blood flow. Yet two months later I was indeed pregnant and gave birth nine months later to a healthy baby boy." Pearl's grandmother used to tell her stories of Indian women who also had a light cream discharge once a month but still became pregnant. Their diet consisted of mainly fruits and vegetables.

Chinese studies show that the first blood flow is closely tied to childhood nutrition. The more fat and protein consumed, the earlier the blood flow begins. American girls start bleeding around the age of twelve, whereas Chinese girls start between the ages of fifteen and nineteen. Although the Chinese girls who eat fast foods and high protein diets start developing their first bleeding at age twelve. Thus verifying that the age of the first bleeding is related to diet and health. We should be concerned about the first blood flow age because studies have shown that early bleeding is related to as high as a ten percent greater risk of breast cancer later in life.

Athletes are considered to be the healthiest people in our society. They run faster jump higher, see better, and throw farther than other humans on this planet. Why then do women athletes stop their monthly blood flow? Modern science says that their low body fat is the reason. My thinking is they are too healthy to have this periodic blood flow. Even if they don't eat a perfect diet, their physical activities protect them from toxins. They get rid of the toxins by either sweating them out though the skin or breathing them out through the lungs. I called T.C. Fry, an author of many books on raw food diets, to ask him about menstruation.

He said, "Don't get menstruation and blood flow mixed up. They are different. Menstruation occurs in healthy women even though the blood goes away. The best people to study to confirm this would be athletes and women who eat raw food."

IS MENSTRUATION NECESSARY?

(Wendy Harris and Nadine Forrest MacDonald)

If many women enjoy good health for a long and happy life, bear several healthy children and never menstruate once in their lives, the least that can be said from these facts is that there is no normal or physiological necessity for the loss of blood each month.

ENDING THE FEMALE "CURSE"

(Victoria Bidwell, reprinted from *Health Seekers Year Book*)

It usually comes as a great shock of disbelief when The Female Health Seeker hears that—with Hygienic living, her "monthly curse" will come to an end! While we can readily understand that sickness and pain will disappear with a program of Natural Hygiene, women deeply steeped in tradition somehow believe that they deserve their monthly bloodletting and its accompanying suffering. Two deep-seated myths, both supported by the medical world, shroud The Menstrual Mentality: first, that the process is a discharge of "impure blood" that prepared the womb for conception; secondly, that the process is essential for and a sign of the woman's fruitfulness. Both myths are entirely erroneous. Women Hygienists have proven, time and again, that they can be "curse-free"—and highly fertile—simultaneously!

...Menstruation is a monthly occurrence in unhealthy females; and it varies in duration and intensity, accordingly. Within a few months of Hygienic living, the blood flow usually dwindles to a day or 2 (or even an hour or 2!) of very light bleeding—with no warning, no pain or aching whatsoever. With strict Hygienic living and when the woman has reached a state of full bodily detoxification, the bleeding stops entirely. And that Dear Woman

Health Seeker, is truly..."a healthy life, LIBERTY, and happiness—pursued and found!!!"

Arnold Ehret wrote in the early 1900's about the benefits of eating a raw vegetarian food diet. He said in his book, *Mucusless Diet Healing System,*

If the female body is perfectly clean through this diet, the menstruation disappears. In scripture it is called by the significant word "purification" which in fact it is clean, no longer polluted by the monthly flow of impure blood and other wastes. Every one of my female patients reported their menses as becoming less and less, then a two, three and four month's intermission, and finally entirely disappearing. This latter condition was experienced by those who went through a perfect cleansing process by this diet.

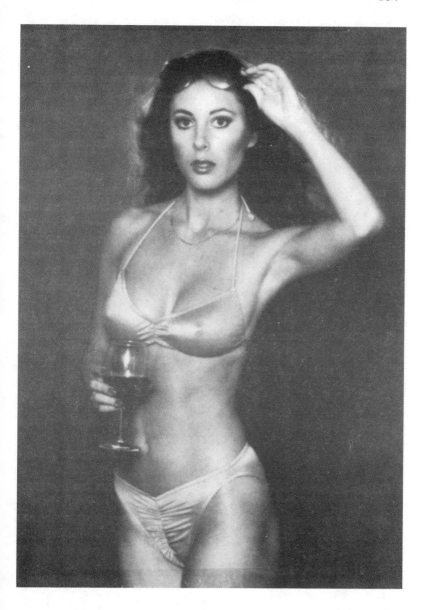

Age 21   Weight: 105 pounds on a meat-eating diet.

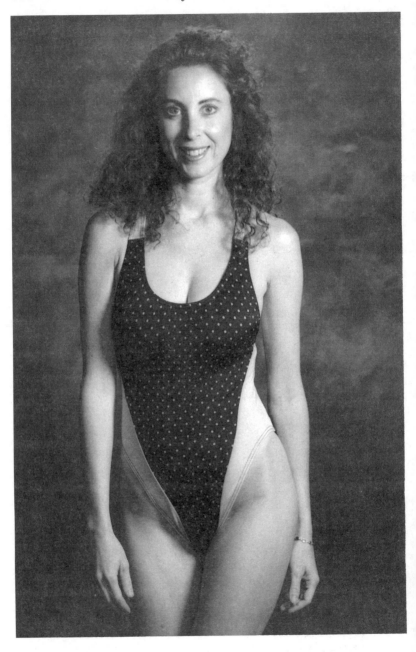

1993 Age 33   Weight: 105 pounds on a vegetarian diet.

19

PREGNANCY AND CHILDREN

My second pregnancy was much easier than my first one because my new diet had strengthened my body tremendously. I had no back pains or muscle cramps. Morning sickness only happened when I strayed from the better diet. Iron during pregnancy was a concern because I was told your iron drops later on in pregnancy and could hurt the baby. I interviewed vegetarian women who had low iron counts to see how they raised their count. Each one tried vitamins fortified with iron first, but this did not work. When they tried leafy green vegetables like Kale soup, Romaine, etc., however, that did work. I ate more grapefruit, watermelon and leafy greens and in my pregnancy I actually increased my iron count to a higher level than the beginning of my pregnancy. People who observed me predicted that the baby I carried was going to be small, since I was not gaining a lot of weight. For instance, at nine months I carried no excess fat or water and my weight gain was only 11 pounds. Perhaps conclusions about low weight pregnancies are wrong because they have been based on non-optimally healthy women such as drug abusers or alcoholics. Not that I was unusual, I interviewed many women who ate better diets and all had small weight gains and very easy child births. Also, their babies scored very high points at birth and midwifes were able to tell which women had healthy diets by the ease of the child's birth.

In her book *Natures Children,* Juliette de Bairachi Levy writes, "During the prenatal month's a women's body must be kept slim and hard in order to prevent formation of a big burdensome child, which will, from its unnatural size, make for difficult child birth and ruin beyond recovery the figure of the mother."

I never held back in eating, yet my body knew what to do with a healthy diet. Baby John was born on August 26, 1992. He took three hours to deliver and weighed in at 6 1/2 pounds. The midwife in the Kaiser hospital in Los Angeles liked the fact that I had researched child birth and realized that I did all the work. She only had to catch the baby. I asked not to be given any drugs and not to have them break my water bag; therefore, Johnny was born with the water sack around him. This turned out to be cleaner and easier for the baby. We did not have Johnny circumcised even though most boys in the USA are circumcised. I wanted to keep the baby the way god created him. The baby and I were so healthy after the birth that we wanted to leave the hospital right away. But hospitals have rules where they must watch the baby for 24 hours before releasing. So we stayed the night. I had no night sweats and was able to walk around immediately.

During the first year of baby John's life, he has only been to the doctor one time. This was for an eye infection, pink eye; however, the antibiotics prescribed for him did not work, so we went to a homeopathic doctor. The homeopathic eye drop remedy worked wonderfully.

When I think back about how I fed my first child on man-made baby formulas and baby food, I realize how influenced we are by big business. If we only could see the big picture and see how diet affects children's health, simple things like ear infections would be unheard of.

We must realize that human milk is very important during the first year of life. Once we choose to go into other foods for the baby, we break the natural blueprint that human milk offers.

Food	Protein Content
	(grams)
4 oz of human milk	2.56
1 banana	1.6
100g of broccoli	3.6
100g of carrot	1.1
10 almonds	18.6
1 small chicken	56.0

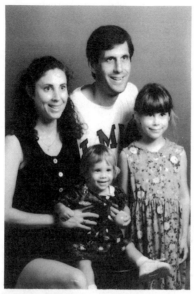

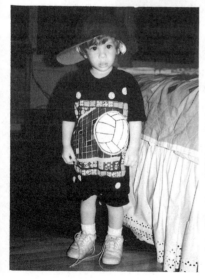

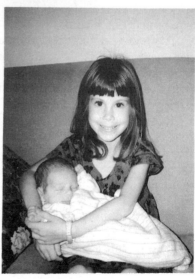

John Olive, 1 Year
John is completely breast fed.

Jacky Olive, Age 6
John Olive, 2 weeks

Lets look at fat content of human milk—

Substance	Fat content (grams)
4 oz of human milk	10.8
1 carrot	0.2
1 orange	0.4
1/2 of an avocado	16.0
1 cup of almonds	26.0
1/2 cup of chickpeas	4.8
4 oz of beef	25.0

You see how easy it would be to reach the necessary fat consumption from a vegetarian diet.

We need to open our eyes and look at what the science of health and nutrition says. Who are you going to trust, mother nature or a lab? Are we to go along with man-made rules and dietary laws that imply man can make better food than nature when illness is so prevalent? Good luck trying to feed your baby one hundred fifty cups of mothers milk a day to get the requirement for niacin.

A good way to teach your child the difference between man-made and mother nature-made food is to look at shapes. Man-made food comes in distinct packages while mother nature foods have imperfect shapes (such as apples, bananas, carrots, etc.).

Researchers at the hospital of the University of Pennsylvania have found that bifidobacteria levels have dropped. Declining bifidobacteria levels may be a result of increased air, water and soil pollution, as well as, increased pesticide and antibiotic use, according to Jeremiah Rasic, Ph.D., and international expert on bifidobacteria.

The bifidobacteria protects babies and young children against a slew of intestinal infections including food poisoning, intestinal disease, aids in vitamin and mineral absorption, weight gain and helps inhibit the growth of disease producing bacteria and yeast.

The importance of organic food is as important to our health as to the baby's.

In Tracy Hotchner's book, *Pregnancy and Childbirth,* she writes, "A totally vegetarian diet may be an excellent way to reduce residues in your system if you start it well enough in advance of breast-feeding. A French study published in 1974 sampled the milk of women who were primarily vegetarians. The results showed that if 70 percent or more of the diet contained organic food (i.e., food grown without synthetic chemical pesticides or fertilizers) the pesticides in the breast milk were less than one-half of those in the median French human milk samples."

People do not understand how to create natural baby food derived from natural sources.

Human milk has a high-fat, low protein content. This is believed necessary to provide enough calories and to aid in the absorption of small quantities of iron. However, even when the ratio is similar, the composition of the protein and fat is usually different. The protein in human milk is primarily lactalbumin which is easily digested by infants, the protein in formula is primarily casein which is not as easily digested.

Sucrose plays a significant role in tooth decay, whereas lactose does not. Studies have shown that children who were breast-fed for 3 months or more had 46 percent fewer cavities during the first 6 years of life than bottle-fed infants—which may be related to the lactose instead of sucrose in their diets. The body metabolizes lactose to galactose, which in turn forms galactolipid, substances which are essential for brain development. Sucrose does not have that benefit.

Mineral content: Human milk contains lower levels of minerals, which minimizes the load on the baby's kidneys.

If the diet the government recommends is correct, why are we so afraid of virus, molds and germs? Why do all our friend's children have ear infections, bronchitis, and colds one after the other?

20

VACCINATIONS

We thought we left the Dark ages behind when our ancestors stopped having kings dictate their children's lives. If the ruler said death to the first born boy, they did as they were told. Could it be that dictators are still alive and operating? Consider immunization. It is one of the dirtiest, sickest, and deadliest things we have done to our children. And again we follow the dictates of powerful leaders such as doctors and pharmaceutical companies and allow our beloved children to be injured by needles which inject filth into them when they are perfectly healthy.

"Most parents and many health care providers do not know that the pertussis (whooping cough) portion of the DPT shot can cause convulsions, shock, brain inflammation, and death. One large US study found that 1 in 875 DPT shots produces a convulsion or collapse/shock reaction, which means that 18,000 DPT shots cause American children to suffer one of these neurological reactions every year."[1]

Instead of just killing the newborn we may be maiming our children because we fear germs.

"Polio had started its decline long before the Salk vaccine made its first appearance."

"No epidemics have occurred in the United states since 1954."[2]

"All cases of paralytic polio in this country since 1979 were either caused by the oral vaccine or contracted in a foreign country during travel. During the period 1980-1985, 55 cases of paralytic polio were reported. Of these cases, 51

---

[1] DPT Brochure, They had no Voice...They had no Choice, 128 Branch Road, Vienna, VA 22180.

[2] Randall Neustaedter, *The Immunization Decision.*

were caused by the vaccine and 4 occurred in people returning from developing countries."[1]

Most diseases run their course and die out. Is this the case today? It appears that we may be bringing back diseases. Doctors see strong and healthy children who never have been sick a day in their life develop illnesses after being given immunization shots.

What are vaccines made from? Materials from which vaccines, serums and biological agents are produced include[2]:

1. Horse blood (for diphtheria toxin and antitoxin)
2. Sweepings from vacuum cleaners (for asthma and hay fever).
3. Pus from sores on diseased animals.
4. Metallic poisons.
5. Powdered insects.
6. Mucus from throats of children with colds and whooping cough.
7. Decomposed fecal matter of typhoid patients.
8. Bacteria.

Are you aware that you are unknowingly electing to inject poisonous bacteria into your child's blood starting at the age of two months? For example:

Age	Bacteria Intake
2 mos.	DTP (diphtheria, tetanus, pertussis) Hib, meningitis, polio, trivalent, OPV#1
4 mos.	repeat the above
6 mos.	DPT#3, Hib.
15 mos.	MMR(measles, mumps, live rubella), DPT#4, Hib, polio, OPV#3
18 mos.	hemophilus influenza B-polysaccharide antigen conjugated to a protein carrier HPCV
4-6 years	DPT#5, Hib, polio, MMR, OPV#4, Mantoux TB
14-16 years	tetanus, diphtheria

---

[1] Ibid.
[2] Hannah Allen, *Don't Get Stuck,* pp.iv, 7, 22, 115.

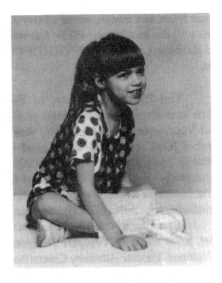

Laura Meyer

Laura was permanently injured by a DPT shot as an infant and Laura was awarded compensation for her injuries under the National Vaccine Injury Compensation Act of 1986 (PL 99-660).

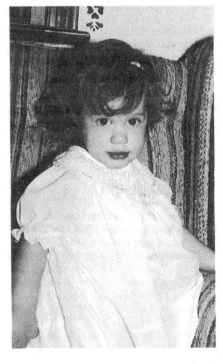

Anna

In January 1989, Anna had her 1st MMR vaccination at 15 months of age. Within two days, she began limping. Over the next two weeks she stopped walking, developed unusual cold symptoms, a 102 degree fever, and was irritable, wanting to be held constantly. Over the next six weeks, she became totally paralyzed. At three years old, Anna cannot walk independently or talk. She is severely handicapped and language delayed.

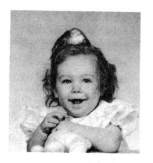

Ashley, May 1991

18 months old
4th DPT & OPV & HIB
Reaction: Within 72 hours, 103
degree fever, lethargy. Hospitalized with kidney failure and en-
cephalitis. **Severely mentally and
physically handicapped.**

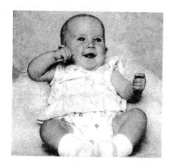

Kimberlie, April 1989

2 months old
1st DPT & OPV
Reaction: Within 3 hours, 103
degree fever, high pitched scream-
ing, convulsions.
**Died: August 1991 of cardiac
arrest**

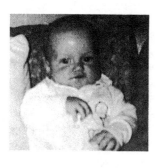

Matthew, January 1990

4 months old
1st DPT & OPV
Reaction: Within 12 hours, pro-
jectile vomiting, staring, behavior
change, very tranquil.
Died: Within 26 hours

Taken from National Vaccine Information Center operated by
Dissatisfied Parents Together, 512 W. Maple Avenue, #206,
Vienna, VA 22180, (703) 938-DPT3, 1-800-909-SHOT.

Who would create such disorder?

"Pasteur was a chemist and physicist, and knew very little about biology and life processes, but he was a respected and influential man. His fear of infection, his belief in the malignity and belligerence of germs, and his powerful influence on his contemporaries, had such far-reaching consequences, that men of science were convinced of the threat of the microbe to man. Thus was born the period of bacteriophobia, germ fear, which still exists."

But in 1880 Pasteur reversed his position, acknowledging that germs are not the specific and primary cause of disease. "It is frequently overlooked that Pasteur by then had changed his direction, and that his more mature conception of the cause of disease was that a germ was ordinarily kept within bounds by natural laws, but, when conditions change, when its virulence is exalted, when its host is enfeebled, the germ was able to invade the territory which was barred to it up to that time. This is, of course, the premise that a healthy body is resistant to disease."[1]

Long ago mankind blamed illness on demons. Today we blame disease on germs. Perhaps neither reason is correct.

Some researchers are finding that the body produces electrical vibrations at variable frequencies. Maybe tuning up body vibrations by eating good foods and surrounding it with wholesome conditions may strengthen it's life force. Let's start with the premise that the God-given body is created perfect! It is humans who create disease by not balancing the five senses.

For those who are looking for a legal way to help stop your child from receiving shots, here's what I did. I wrote away for an affidavit for exemption from school inoculation.

[1] Ibid.

21

OLD AGE

Accepting the fact that we are growing old may be the scariest fact one has to face. Most people try desperately to avoid admitting it. They surgically remove wrinkles and fat, transplant hair, go on diets, do face makeovers, and talk about not growing old. Some would rather die then grow old. No one wants to spend any time thinking about old age.

What is aging and why does it occur? Why do some people age faster than others? Are questions about it unanswerable?

Look at man's history. In the beginning of the Bible we find people live to be hundreds of years old.

"And all the days that Adam lived were nine hundred and thirty years; and he died.

"And all the days of Seth were nine hundred and twelve years; and he died.

"And all the days of Enosh were nine hundred and five years and he died.

"And all the days of Kenan were nine hundred and ten years and he died.

"And all the days of Mahalate were eight hundred and five years and he died.

"And all the day of Noah were nine hundred and fifty years and he died."

After Noah and the flood, people began to eat animals. Thereafter, people's life spans were shorter.

"And the days of Terah were two hundred and five years; and Terah died in Haran.

"And the days of Isaac were a hundred and fourscore years. And Isaac expired, and died, and was gathered unto his people, old and full of days.

"So Joseph died, being a hundred and ten years old.

"And the years of the life of Levi were a hundred thirty and seven years.

"And Moses was a hundred and twenty years old when he died."

The Bible records history of ancient peoples. Many modern people will tell you these life numbers are wrong, but that's just opinions because truly no one knows why we age. As a matter of fact, when scientists look closely at our molecules they say our bodies are designed to live longer lives than we are achieving. We see in nature that wild animals live long lives:

Animal	Approximate life (years)
Eagles	500
Turtles	500
Parrots	600-700
Wild hogs	300

My point is this. Many people don't want to grow old because of the fear of disease. They just don't have the knowledge on how to grow old healthfully. If they would treat their bodies as temples of God, they would have a much longer healthier life span.

In the *Hunza of the Himalayas,* Renee Taylor writes about the Hunza's secrets of long life and happiness. I also spoke with two medical doctors (P. Joyalakshi and K.R. Sampathas) who lived with the Hunzas and verified their longevity. Maybe the following are their secrets?

1. The Hunza people keep active until the day they die.

2. They don't think about clocks or calendars.

3. They don't retire-one must never retire "from" something. One must retire "to" something.

4. They have no rest homes because a person needs a sense of belonging just as a plant will die if it is placed in an alien and infertile soil.

5. They are cheerful and enjoy work.

6. They meditate.

7. Their goal is to create a balance of mind and body.

8. They practice sensible living-natural remedies instead of medical treatment.

9. They work slowly.

10. They pray twice a day. Every muscle and nerve is relaxed during their prayers.

11. They rest between tasks even if only a few minutes.

12. They use no electricity, kerosene, or candles. They are obliged to retire early and rise early. They happily accept their way of life.

13. Their diet is very close to nature. They eat lots of fruit (such as cherries, apricots, grapes, mulberries, apples, pears, peaches), vegetables (raw lettuce, carrots, sprouted parsley, squash, spinach, turnip, peas, beans, radishes, potatoes), grains (whole wheat, buckwheat, rice millet), cottage cheese yogurt, herb tea, apricot oil, and on rare occasions meat. Any heating of food is done on low flame. The fruit and vegetables are completely ripened on the tree or vine before they eat them.

14. Children are treated with courtesy and they return the same to the adults.

15. Everyone drinks an abundance of water which is not boiled or filtered. The water is rich in minerals which gives it a grey color called glacial milk. And is drunken straight from the streams.

16. They chant the mantra sound "ommmmomommmmm".

17. They work and play outdoors in the fresh air.

18. They grind their own grain immediately when they harvest it.

19. They use no yeast or baking soda in their breads, instead they use chapatti which is made from whole wheat flour water. They bake their bread slowly on low heat.

20. Their organic agriculture system supports a large population. They use terraced fields located on mountainsides.

21. They have no jails because they have no crime.

22. They have no banks because they have no money.

23. They are mostly farmers, cooks, mountain porters, tailors, gold smiths, and weavers.

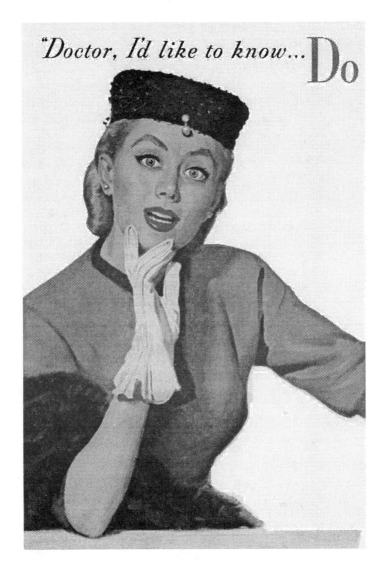

"*Doctor, I'd like to know...* Do

24. As a rule, no one owns more than five acres of land which is enough for one family's needs.

25. If something happens to a villager, all the neighbors stand by to offer a helping hand.

26. Education is free to all.

I have to grow old?¨

No, not as your grandparents or even your parents did. The doctors have learned in recent years that there is much that can be done to help make all of life's years happy and productive.

They have learned that a zest for living, a liking for people, serenity of spirit, peace of mind, sensible living and eating, all are important. They now know that good eating habits in particular have a vital learing on the retention of physical vigor, mental alertness and, above all, the protection of the heart, the arteries, the glandular system and the digestive tract.

Your doctor will tell you that a diet based upon the generous use of such protective foods as fresh fruits and leafy vegatables not only helps to keep you healthy but has a lot to do with keeping your physical stamina and mental alertness "young"!

At any age the protective foods should be used generously in the daily diet. Among the best, as we grow older, are bananas, because of their easy digestibility, because they do not require vigorous chewing, because they supply needed vitamins and minerals, because they are effective in weight control, and because they have such a beneficent effect on the entire digestive system.

Why not eat to add life to your years as well as to add years to your life.

Because of the many appetizing ways in which bananas can be served, as well as because of their importance in nutrition, bananas are now being used more widely than ever by people of all ages.

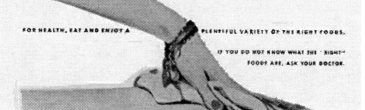

FOR HEALTH, EAT AND ENJOY A PLENTIFUL VARIETY OF THE RIGHT FOODS.

IF YOU DO NOT KNOW WHAT THE 'RIGHT' FOODS ARE, ASK YOUR DOCTOR.

27. No disease.

28. They fast in late spring when there is no food for them.

29. All food is grown organically.

30. What the Hunza take out of the earth they put back. Cattle manure, vegetable parts, fallen leaves and ashes are

mixed together to form compost and spread over the fields.

31. Old age is not feared because the Hunza do not die a horrid painful death. They die many times in their sleep at ages over 100.

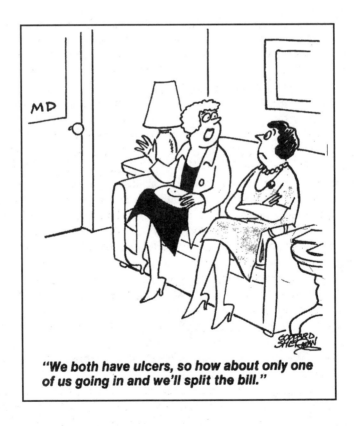

"We both have ulcers, so how about only one of us going in and we'll split the bill."

22

DOCTORS

How does this sound? *Kick the Disease Habit.* Join a club we can all belong to. It's purpose? To educate ourselves. Sounds like a good idea to me. Just think what would happen to the insurance rates. Why not have more information for the public on health problems?

But in some places in America, it is illegal to give information for people on healing and disease. The medical, pharmaceutical and nutritional field has tried to monopolize the health field. Most doctors treat with the knowledge that they were taught in school: drugs and surgery. Nutritionists were taught a standard textbook laboratory system.

In the old days, when a child was sick, the doctor gave him the best medicine for what ailed him. Today they don't do that. They give him what is commercially available... something good for ten thousand people cannot be good for one man.

We are allowed to run our houses, cars, and businesses, but when it comes to our bodies we have been kept in the dark. Why can't we mass educate ourselves on the house of our bodies? I have a brain, too, and can learn how to run my own house.

Many in the medical field think that anyone who treats differently is wrong—just like a lot of religions. If people want to choose what clothes they wear, what food they eat, what religion they practice, they surely can pick what form of healing they want. Why should our government stop the way we choose to heal ourselves?

Instead, the government should work for the people to get more information on foods and herbs, and to teach us about the mind-body connection.

The government and doctors feel they are protecting their citizens by only giving one choice, doctors or nutritionists, who are trained in the same information. Yet they let people sell poison: cigarettes, alcohol, chemicals, drugs (aspirin, Tylenol, etc.), milk, etc. We are subconsciously told in advertisements how were going to be healthier if we eat these chemicals. These businesses are not put in jail for outright lying to the public.

Because it is a freedom of choice country, if you want to poison yourself go ahead, but if you want health advice there is only one way, drugs and surgery. No wonder our country has a drug problem.

In the book, *The Tao of Medicine,* Dr. Stephen Fulder writes: "The Harmony remedies seemed to affect all the major body functions. It was beyond belief. Then I stepped back from science and suddenly realized that the river is like the flow of energy in the whole being, and all the scientific material seemed to be like efforts to cut this river into small ponds of water."

"It is time the field of medicine looked at itself for what it is. In my opinion their science is a science of unknowing ignorance. They cut and burn the poisons out with drugs before they try to balance the energy field. Because they have no understanding of the auric field, MD's do not comprehend the side effects of their drugs. They do not realize that the new diseases of Rhyes Syndrome, Alzheimer's, and Aids may be products of their inability to understand the electromagnetic balancing of the curaic field."[1]

Look at the Chernobyl accident of 1986. Within one year of the toxins being released, it has created many malformations in humans and animals.

Writing in the Philadelphia Inquirer on January 14, 1990, Steve Goldstern reports, "The first news that something strange was happening in Narodichi came in the fall of 1988 as rumors swirled in Kiev about illnesses among children and the birth of defected animals."

"People still live in these contaminated areas."

---

[1] Dean Hardy, Mary Hardy, Marjorie, Killick, Kenneth Killick, *Pyramid Energy, The Philosophy of God, The Science of Man,* pp.206-208, 212, 213.

"I grow potatoes and apples. Maybe I can live without apples but how can I live without potatoes? My pigs eat the same things. Is it dangerous? What else can we do? We live here and it grows here. I don't know what will be the future for us."

For Ugana and her friends, the danger of radiation is neither clear nor present in their minds—it's not something they can see, smell or comprehend. "The milk was white, and now it is still white," they say."

"We have lived with radiation for three years, and we don't care anymore—when our time comes, we will die, and the cows will die, too. I'm 71, and me and my husband have been living here for 55 years. I won't go away. I will stay here in my corner and wait until I die. We have a place under the birch tree down there."

This is the same attitude right here in United States. They are disgusted with what's going on and don't know how to help. They are confused and sit back and figure everything will be all right. Besides, I'll be dead in 20 years and I won't see the mess we left behind.

"Studies on radiation on the body links to heart disease, nervous-system disorders, cancer, immune damage...In other studies small doses of the radiation stimulate the immune system. "The residents of Kiev and near Chernobyl reported a decline in the incidence of common colds."

People do not understand the function of the common cold which is cleansing the toxins out of the body. If the body has illness and cannot catch a cold this is devastating to the cleansing system as it must rid itself of bacteria.

The basic concept of chemotherapy is so toxic that the patient's hair falls out completely and will not grow back for six months. They become extremely nauseous and throw up from chemotherapy. Then they form other immune weaknesses.

Yet, sometimes, the tumor shrinks. Could the body be so full of toxins from radiation that it stops forming the tumor to protect other bodily functions? In reality, the tumor was a good sign telling the person that something was wrong. It seals off the toxins into one lump to protect the body from the harmful toxins. By giving the body radiation, it cannot protect you any longer. Instead of radiation helping, could the procedure be speeding up death? The recovery rate between chemotherapy and cutting the cancer out is no different. The doctors just don't see the whole picture.

A patient with cancer goes into the hospital and instead of feeding him Jell-O for breakfast, the nurse will squeeze fresh juice served within minutes to make sure all the nutrients are fresh and the enzymes are alive. We will put them through a complete nutrition program before resorting to alternative methods.

We in the West are probably the most pain-conscious people on the face of the earth. For years we have been conditioned—in print, on radio, over television, in daily conversation—that any hint of pain is to be banished as though it were the ultimate evil. Consequently we become pill-grabbers and hypochondriacs, escalating the slightest headache into a searing ordeal. Dangerously, pain-killing drugs conceal pain without correcting the underlying condition. Our bodies can pay a high price for this suppression without regard to its basic cause. When we develop pain, anxiety, depression, or any of a host of physical symptoms, it is nature's way of telling us to pay attention to some neglected aspect of our lives. (From *Inner Health* by Nevill Drury (p. 48).

There are many ways to strengthen the immune system to fight disease.

We will see a high percentage of disease fought by following a health maintenance program.

HEALTH MAINTENANCE PROGRAM

1. Eating a complete raw diet. Make sure the digestion is slowly built up to learn fast energy of raw food. Cook foods until digestion is stronger.
2. Follow human mother's milk as a comparison for protein, fat, sugar and minerals. Fruit should be eaten breakfast and dinner. Vegetables for lunch or fruit all day. Zucchini and cucumber are fruits.
3. Follow digestion time of food.
4. Follow food combining.
5. Do not overeat, only 1 to 2 pieces of fruit per meal.

6. Make sure you are hungry when eating. Follow breakfast lunch and dinner schedule: 8:30 - 12:00 - 5:00.
7. Fasting breakfast or holding out in the morning until very hungry. This way body can eat up bacteria. Fasting when strong enough.
8. Rotate diet.
9. Make sure all color of food is in diet.
10. Add whole herb foods. Cell cleansing formulas, cell building, acidophilus.
11. Add nuts and seeds in small amounds. Almond milk or other nut milk drinks-all raw. Do not eat too many high protein or high sugar raw foods.
12. Learn Yin and Yang of foods. Sweet and bitter foods at one meal for balance.
13. Go to bed early - 9:00 or 10:00 - get up with the sun.
14. Do not eat before sleeping - body needs to rebuild, not digest food. Follow digestion time of food.
15. Learn body cycles—cleansing: 5:00 am to 12:00 noon; Nourishment: 12:00 noon to 7:00 pm; Assimilation: 7:00 pm to 5:00 am
16. Sunshine one hour a day with no sunglasses.
17. Exercise by walking.
18. Clean food well so there is no visible bacteria on it.
19. All food eaten should be organically grown.
20. Make sure you eat the whole food, fiber and all.
21. Blend foods for soups.
22. Yoga.
23. Massage body.
24. Meditate.
25. Use color therapy.
26. Sound therapy.
27. Aromatherapy.
28. Use principles of earth, air, fire, water elements. *
29. Colonics.
30. Breathing Exercises

*Earth: touching, smelling and becoming one with earth.
 Air: learning deep breathing exercises.
 Water: cleaning in showers or baths 1-2 times a day.
 Fire: sitting by a fire to cleanse the spiritual body.

HEAVEN'S GROCERY STORE

*I was walking down life's
 highway,
A long time ago.
One day I saw the sign that
 read,
"Heaven's Grocery Store."
As I got a little closer,
The door came open wide;
And when I came to myself,
I was standing inside.
I saw a host of angels,
They were standing
 everywhere.
One handed me a basket, and
 said,
"My child, shop with care."
Everything a person needed
Was in that grocery store.
And all you couldn't carry,
You could come back the next
 day for more.
First I got some Patience,
Love was in the same row.
Farther down was Under-
 standing,
You need that wherever you
 go.
I got a box or two of
 Wisdom;
A bag or two of Faith.
I couldn't miss the Spirit,
For it was all over the place.
I stopped to get some
 Strength
and Courage
To help me run this race.
By then my basket was
 getting full,*

*But I remembered I needed
 some Grace.
I didn't forget Salvation,
For Salvation is free;
So I tried to get enough
 of that
To save both you and me.
Then I started to go up to the
 counter,
To pay my grocery bill,
For I thought I had enough
Of everything
To do my Master's will.
As I went up the aisle, I
 saw Prayer,
And I just had to put that in,
For I knew that when I
 stepped
outside,
I would run right into Sin.
Peace and Joy were plentiful,
They were on the last shelf.
Song and Praise were hanging
 near,
So I just helped myself.
Then I said to the angel,
"Now how much do I owe?"
He just smiled and said,
"Just take them everywhere
 you go."
Again I smiled and said,
"How much do I really owe?"
He smiled and said,
"My child, the Good lord paid
 your bill,
     A long time ago."*

- Author Unknown

23

FUTURE

"Imagine this. One morning you awaken from a peaceful sleep. As you lie on your organically grown, cotton futon, with its naturally dyed crimson red silk sheets, your room, of wooden construction, emits a fragrance...combining the sweet, natural smells of the aromatic woods...and where the wood is covered, an almost sensual aroma of citrus-based plant paints.

"You rise and glide across a natural, toxin-free plush carpet. The sun, shining through the many skylights, makes your bare skin feel really nice. Each room is filled with light and life, including a profusion of green and flowering plants. The skylights are laced with solar panels, perhaps in some significant spiritual mandala, generating heat and electrical energy.

"You turn on the sun heated shower; whose pristine waters have passed through a simple diatomaceous filtration system.

"Stepping out of your comfortable, natural-fiber sandals, the clean warm water showers your naked body; tingling and caressing your skin as you splash on a natural plant-based skin cleanser. A natural lemon oil water rinse, a quick sun dry, and perhaps a brief meditation.

"The walls around you are pure, no artificial toxins or radiation from the materials or from the small amount of electrical wiring inside the walls, shielded from emitting questionable electromagnetic waves..." This was written by SW. Nostradamus Virato in the *New Frontier* magazine (Philadephia, PA).

We have lived on this planet for thousands of years with no problem with pollution, so the best thing to do is study people who were successful in developing civilizations that worked.

"The Hohokans lived in Arizona. They had a canal system. The canals stretched for miles along the upper terrace of the river valley, safe from sudden floods yet near at hand for maintenance and water control and for directing water in the fields. The canals were well planned and executed which led to centuries of peace and prosperity.

"After so many years of association with the vanished Hohokans, I am convinced that their achievement is instructive for our own time. Their secret of success was profoundly simple. They came to grips with, but did not abuse, nature. They became a part of the ecological balance instead of destroying it. They accepted the terms of their existence in a difficult environment, and they continued for well over 1,000 years.

"For our own generation, with its soiled streams and fouled air, its massive and abrupt changes in environment, its shortages of water, its rampant misuse of shrinking open space, the achievement of Snaketown holds a profound meaning."[1]

Think of how long humans have been living in harmony with nature. For more than 8000 years we used all things in wholes.

We can help companies change by giving them ideas to create live and whole food products. Once people realize the benefit of better foods we will see an increase of enzymes on the package just as we have done with fiber. Labels will state the enzyme content in the package.

Our Doctors, will learn the healing power of whole food. Our hospitals will have whole foods only because a hospital is for the out-of-balance body. One day there will be no names for disease because the body is actually out-of-balance. Set up at the front desk of the hospital will be a food dictionary which will inform the public which foods will strengthen the body. All books will be open to the public.

You will be able to recognize the people of the future quickly. They will have correct posture because of yoga, the skin will be baby soft because of a high fruit diet; there will be no need for sunglasses; there will be an increased use of solar energy; people will grow long hair; the whites of our eyes will show no yellow and the eye color will have no brown spots.

---

[1]   Emil W. Haury, *National Geographic*, May 1967.

The muscles in our bodies will be strong from working the earth.

One day there will be college courses offering this information.

Mother nature won't allow her lands to be stripped, poisoned and electrified without a fight. A fight noble and powerful. The people who realize the changes needed will become strong and directed. The people who won't change with nature will become sickly and weak.

There will be a new race of people. A people who will live for tomorrow and for today; a people who will live in harmony with nature. They will be a hard-working people who won't mind helping in any chance they get. They will clean up the mess the others leave behind.

These people will understand nature and what is happening. They will be able to look around at the suffering and know it is their choice because they didn't listen. And yet, there will be a kindness in their heart that always forgives and teaches the correct principles when ready.

So what are the correct principles? We try to make life so difficult by our silly high technology, yet life is so simple. Natural energy is available everywhere you look.

Sun-solar	Rocks
Wheel	Wood
Magnetic	Leaves
Sand	Human power
Clay	Animal power
Weight-heavy/light	Water
God	

God is the most available energy there is. There are a few people in our past, as well as right now, who know how to use God's vibrational energy. The more we concentrate on what man wants in a man-made world, the further we get from God's world, the more we will destroy our planet.

Change the energy: you change the manifestation of the mass.

By studying light energy, we free ourselves from man's world and raise ourselves back towards God's world.

We must study and learn from the great teachers how to change our energy to one that is compatible with the earth.

Nikola Tesla discovered light energy, tachion energy, and rotating magnetic fields. He was born in 1856 on the Austrian-Hungarian border and arrived in America with his knowledge in 1884.

"Tesla's great gift to mankind was the understanding of light, and tachion energy. In fact he developed a device called a tachiometer, that measured the pulsed energy. He took light apart frequency by frequency. He could magnify its pulsed output, his AC Theory. He could put this knowledge into the laboratory situation and give mankind the technology of electricity we have today. There isn't an electrical motor running today that isn't using one of Tesla's patents."[1]

All Tesla's books on light can not be bought in the United States. Light energy would have been free, with no pollution, so no one profits from it, so no one wanted his ideas.

The Indians also knew about light energy. Remembering the rain dances, this was done with vibrational patterns through chants and dance. Sound and movement changes the vibrations and you change the weather.

There were mysterious Indian schools to learn light energy. Here the Indians were taught the secrets of vibration through dancing, drumming and chanting.

Indian healers were called shamans. They, as well, knew how to change the energy. The Navajo medicine men performed healing energies which harmonized with the vibrations of chanting, color, light, herbs and fumigants.

[1] Pyramid Energy, The Philosophy of God, The Science of Man by Dean Hardy, Mary Hardy, Marjorie Killick, Kenneth Killick, pp.206-208, 212, 213.

"The Navajo are firmly convinced that the flow of energy moves freely through the Earth, and through all living things, and that to benefit from these, one must not disturb the flow, but simply create vibrations that alter flow to be more advantageous."

"When the energy levels are changed by cutting the forest and clearing the land it is necessary to return the energy to balance. Otherwise the water will run off and the area will dry up. The trees are Nature's antennas between the sky and the land. When the energy is balanced, mineralized water is pulled up to the surface by the electrical balance between the Earth and the atmosphere. Nature is first electrical then chemical. We must return to an understanding of the electrical side of Nature."[1]

For Mankind to go back to a natural world he must learn and study nature's forces.

[1] Ibid.

24

THE END

So, you have changed your diet, you feel great, you are regenerating new silky, smooth skin, you are getting younger every year instead of older. There are no more headaches or flu. Life is wonderful, yet something is missing. You are hanging around with the same people who are doing the normal diet. These people want everyone to have the same— same religion, same clothes, same furniture, same doctors...safety in numbers. They talk about the pain they are in, of people dying of heart attacks and of cancer. Their raunchy bad breath reeks of dead food as they tell you of their woe's. The fat around their stomach protrudes ten inches of thick toxins. Their chin jiggles in fat as they eat their cooked, oily foods and puff their cigarettes.

You want to shout and scream about what you found— **THE FOUNTAIN OF LIFE!** But, they stare at you. You don't partake in the ceremonials of food. What's wrong with you? Sickness must be your problem. Sickness is catchy-BEWARE OF MARY! But you tell them NO. There is something wrong with the food. You warn them because you love them and care about their well being.

They shout at you, "THERE'S NOTHING WRONG WITH THE WAY I EAT!"

My father and forefathers always ate this way and they lived to be 85 and that's good enough. You tell them the Pottenger cat story of degeneration with each generation. They want to know who wrote the story and if they had any credentials. Are they doctors? Give me proof. Then, they try to manipulate you by yelling louder to scare you off because they are afraid of change.

You say fine, I only told you because I love you. They say if you are going to talk about this subject, they don't want you around. So, you stop talking and you stop listening to their aches and pains. You stop reading the articles on their made up cancer and the AIDS virus because you know there is no such thing on mother nature's diet. Then you master the art of being indifferent. Indifference is when you love everything and everybody so you let them go. You realize they need to grow and learn at their own pace. Yet, you are always there if you are needed.

I learned the hard way that I was different. I read and read and tried until I found the correct answers. I have found that 95% of our population will not even pick up a book to educate themselves.

In the book, *The Awful Truth about Publishing*, John Boswell writes, "Books sustain the mind, not the body, and are therefore not considered to be one of life's essentials. Sadly, books aren't even a popular form of entertainment. Most Americans read a book only when there is nothing on the tube and no other diversions available to them.

"Ten years ago a blockbuster best seller like *The Godfather* or *The Exorcist* sold twelve million copies. Today a huge best seller sells three million copies—or to about one percent of the population. This is probably the most depressing of the awful truths for people within the publishing industry. Sometimes people who work in publishing feel like all the people who actually buy and read books could fit at one time into the Astrodome."

That is why the truth is not known. Empty brains get empty thoughts.

I asked my husband, John, if he would help me educate people on health. He said, "No I'm a basketball coach. I don't want to help people with health." I said, "I am an artist. If no one wants to help, we will get nowhere. So it had better start with me. Writing a book would be an easier way to help more people and hopefully the information will be passed on to generations."

I am not saying that I am perfect. I am just like the rest. Sometimes I even have a cookie or a brownie, but I do know better and I know where to make changes when I am feeling awful. I take responsibility for my own health. I am not a great writer either, but I can show you experts on every subject I feel is important to health. Remember a collective mind is better than one mind.

The more I think about life the simpler it becomes. We must see everything in a whole working symphony. Nature will start taking over your mind and start teaching you about life.

We know 100 years ago mother earth was clean and beautiful. Mankind's thoughts and actions were not balanced, but because of the earth's cleanness mankind could tolerate cooked foods and imperfect thinking. The cleanness of the earth balanced with mankind's toxicity kept man alive. Now the earth is polluted and mankind is polluted which creates a bigger problem. This is why it is so important that we balance our sense to be able to live on the polluted earth.

Love is the backbone to salvaging the earth. Once we love ourselves, love thy neighbor and go on to love the land, air, water, plants and animals, we will be successful. We must stop thinking about the way we look on the outside and spend more time thinking about the ingredients to make a superior human being, and a healthy plant, the nourishment and love to feed the mother earth.

I was thinking of giving this book to the doctor who told me to go and see a psychiatrist and of how being an artist saved my life, to never limit my mind and always keep ideas open and flowing and discussing how most of the world was wrong by taking things apart and isolating them. I was not crazy, I just did not understand the life process at the time. I would show him how I analyzed the situation myself. I do wonder if he would read the book or if he would think that I was insane. Although when you master the art of indifference you realize—SW, SW, SW—Some will, some won't, so what, next!

May your journey through life bring you higher levels of love and wisdom.

Diane Olive

Appendix 1

RECIPES

The following recipes are provided for people who want to learn to eat from Earth's plate and who want a better future. The recipes are mainly composed of raw foods, but do use some cooked items. Your goal should be to slowly add raw foods to your diet. The recipes give you an opportunity to eat tasty foods and at the same time to bring good nutrition to your body.

John, Jacky and I played with our food until we found a comfortable diet. Our breakfast is fruit, lunch is vegetables, nuts, seeds or grains, and dinner is fruit. Remember, the better nourished you are the less hungry you are. All bodies are different for the nutrients they need.

As the seasons change so does our nutritional needs. Listen to your body and to your own requirements.

Do not eat the same foods over and over again. Once the body has gotten nutrients from a particular food it will not need this food again for awhile. Creating your own rotating diet is the best for your body.

Most recipes are designed for 1-2 people.

BREAKFAST

grapefruit	apples	figs	papaya
grapes	banana	dates	peach
oranges	melons	pears	cherries
strawberries	pineapple	persimmons	apricots
tangerine	grapefruit	blueberries	kiwis

GREAT BREAKFAST

Put whole bananas in bowl then smash. Cut up 2 dates and sprinkle on top of bananas.

APPLE SALAD

Cut up 2 apples, walnuts and add raisins.
Apples can be put through Champion juicer to have an applesauce consistency.

OATMEAL

Soak in water 1/2 of cup oat groats or 1/2 of cup oat flakes over night. Add dates. Cut 4 walnuts in pieces and add 1 tablespoon of sorghum.

LUNCH

By eating the biggest meal at lunchtime it gives you the rest of the day to digest food. This allows a better sleep at night by not having to digest your food, but repairing the body. Make sure your lunch is full of colors and sweet and sour tastes.

SOUPS

SUNFLOWER SOUP

1 Tbsp. of sunflower seeds	1/2 avocado
1 rib of celery	1 carrot
1 small onion	1/2 clove garlic
1/2 Squash (like zucchini)	1/2 cup water

Food process all ingredients and blend. Sprinkle with sunflower seeds in the bowls.

SOUP CHOWDER

1 carrot	1 corn on the cob
1/4 avocado	Basil
1 onion	Sea salt
1 rib of celery	Water to blend

Blend 3/4's of ingredients together and take the remainder and cut small. Add to blended soup.

SPLIT PEA SOUP

1/2 cup split peas - soaked overnight
1 carrot
1 tablespoon flaxseed oil
1/2 squash
1/2 cup water
1 clove garlic

2 ribs of celery
2 leaves Romaine lettuce
1/2 avocado
1/2 onion
1 teaspoon sea salt

Blend all ingredients in the blender.

NOTE: If you are on a transitional diet, cook one-half of the ingredients.

AVOCADO DROP SOUP

1 tablespoon of Braggs
1/2 avocado

2 cups water

Smash the avocado in the mixture of Braggs and water.

CARROT SOUP

2 carrots
1/2 turnip
1 teaspoon celery seed

1/2 avocado
1/2 onion
1 clove garlic

1 teaspoon herbamare herb seasoning salt

Food process 3\4's of ingredients and blend. Take remainder and cut small. Mix with blended soup.

CELERY SOUP

2 ribs of celery
1/2 avocado
Garlic
1 rib of celery

1/4 onion
Basil leaf
Jerusalem artichokes

Blend the first five ingredients. Cut artichokes and celery in small pieces. Combine all ingredients.

BROCCOLI SOUP

1 corn on cob or 1 cup of corn
1/4 avocado

1 cup broccoli
1/4 onion - cut small

Blend broccoli and corn. Top soup with small pieces of cut broccoli, avocado and onions.

TOMATO SOUP

1 large tomato	1/4 Squash
garlic	small onion
1/2 stalk celery	1/2 cup water
oregano	1/4 avocado

Food process all of the above ingredients and add cut up pieces of squash, celery, onions, avocado and tomato.

KALE SOUP

10 leaves of kale	2 leaks
1/2 cup lima beans - frozen	1 cob corn
1 cup rice - soaked overnight	1 carrot
1 cup beans - soaked overnight	1/2 cup peas - frozen
2 teaspoons italian seasoning	3 sticks of celery
1 teaspoon seaweed	

Cook beans and rice for 1/2 hour and add kale and rest of vegetables. Simmer for 45 minutes longer. Serve with bowls of cut-up raw vegetables (celery, carrot, raw corn, peas). Pour soup on top.

MILLET SOUP

1 cup cooked millet	1 carrot
1/4 head of cabbage	1/4 onion
1 celery stick	1/2 cup of water

Blend all raw vegetables in blender. Put a scoop of millet in each bowl. Top with raw vegetable mixture.

SWEET POTATO SOUP

1 large Sweet potato cooked or raw	
1 teaspoon cinnamon	1/2 cup of water

Blend all ingredients.

MAIN DISHES

AVOCADO LETTUCE

1/2 Avocado	Flaxseed powder
Anary Seed	Lettuce leaves
Dulse	

Take 1/2 avocado and sprinkle with dusle, flaxseed powder and powdered anary seeds served on top of lettuce.

CHINESE FOOD - 1

1 carrot	4 mushrooms
20 Cashews	2 ribs of celery
1/2 head lettuce - cut small	1/4 Jicama
1/2 small onion	

Cut all ingredients in small pieces.

Sauce:

1 tablespoon of Braggs or soy sauce
1 clove garlic
small piece of fresh ginger
5 drops of sweetener

Blend all sauce ingredients and combine with above mixture. Serve on a bed of shredded iceberg lettuce.

CHINESE FOOD - 2

1 carrot - sliced	1 squash - sliced
1/4 head of cabbage - sliced	1 rib of celery - sliced
Small piece of onion - chopped small	Romaine lettuce - cut small

Rice (or fresh corn for substitute)

Combine ingredients and serve with China Roll sauce (see following recipe).

CHINA ROLL

2 cups zucchini	1 carrot
1 tablespoon of onion	2 celery sticks cut small
1/4 cup of cashews cut small	1 cup sprouts
1/2 avocado cut small	1/2 cup water
1 cup Cooked millet (optional)	1 tablespoon tamari
1 tablespoon flax seed powder	1/4 cup water
4 sea weed wraps	

Put all vegetable ingredients in food processor. Take the flax seed, tbsp. tamari, 1/2 cup water, avocado and 1/4 cup of vegetable mix and blend to make sauce. Combine with vegetables. Wet the sea weed wraps with a mixture of the tsp. tamari and 1/4 cup water and roll up the vegetable mixture.

TASTER DELIGHT

1 carrot
1 rib of celery
1/2 cup of cabbage
1/2 avocado
Juice of 1/2 lemon
lettuce - cut small
1/4 cup pine nuts

1/4 onion
sprouts
1/4 cup of nori sea weed
1/4 cup water
1 tablespoon flaxseed oil
Nori rolls

Food process vegetables. To prepare sauce take 1/4 cup water, avocado, 1/4 of the vegetables and then add the rest of the vegetables. Use flaxseed oil and lemon juice mist to moisten nori roll. Roll vegetables in nori sheets.

PEAS AND CORN

Lettuce
1/2 cup corn

1/2 cup peas

Mix peas and corn and place on lettuce.

CABBAGE NORI

2 cups cabbage - food process
1/4 cup food processed cabbage
    blended with 1/2 cup avocado
1 tablespoon flaxseed oil
1 teaspoon flaxseed powder
2 teaspoons caraway powder
1/4 cup water

Mix ingredients together.

1 carrot grated
1 cup Alfalfa sprouts - washed well
1 tablespoon plum paste, mixed with 1/4 cup water
1/2 pickle cut into slivers
1 tablespoon sesame butter

4 Nori sheets

Take the nori sheet and spread with plum paste. Put processed cabbage onto middle of sheet. Sprinkle with more plum paste, add sesame butter. Add the grated carrots, pickle, sprouts, more cabbage and then roll.

CINNAMON ROLLS

1 teaspoon cinnamon	1/4 cup raisins
1/8 cup pine nuts	1/4 head white cabbage
1/4 head purple cabbage	1/4 beet
1 small piece of ginger	1/2 avocado
4 Nori sheets	lemon-water

Food process the white and purple cabbage. Take 1/4 of the food processed mixture and blend with cinnamon, avocado, and ginger.

Mix blended ingredients with the remaining food processed cabbage and add the pine nuts and raisins. Mix the juice of 1/2 lemon and water. Use the lemon rind to rub onto the nori sheets to moisten. Fill with vegetables and roll.

BEAN BURRITOS

2 cups pinto beans-cooked or soaked and sprouted

1 tablespoon onion-cut small	1 tomato-cut small
4 mushrooms-cut small	1 carrot-shredded
2 tablespoons of salsa	1/2 avocado

1/2 cup buckwheat sprouts-cut small
Nori wraps or flour tortillas

Grind pinto beans and mix all ingredients. Moisten nori wraps and roll above ingredients in nori wraps.

SALSA

2 tomatoes-cut up small	1/2 onion
1 teaspoon of sea salt or dulse	1/4 cup cilantro
1 clove garlic	

Mix all ingredients in a bowl.

GUACAMOLE

2 avocados - smash with fork	1/2 onion-finely cut
1 tomato-cut small	1/4 cup cilantro

Mix all ingredients together.

CELERY SALAD

2 ribs of celery-cut small	1/4 cup raisins
7 walnuts-cut small	

Mix all ingredients together.

ROMAINE TACOS

1/4 red onion-finely chopped	Broccoli-cut small
1 yellow squash-shredded	1 avocado-cut small
1/2 cup sunflower sprouts-cut small	10 cashews-cut small
4 romaine lettuce leaves	4 mushrooms-cut small

Serve with each vegetable in a pile on plate. Each person fills their own romaine leaf with vegetables.

CHICK PEA SPREAD

1 cup chick peas - soaked overnight	1/4 avocado
1 teaspoon herb seasoning	2 teaspoons dill weed
1/2 water	1/2 zucchini
1/2 cup sesame seeds ground into a powder (use coffee grinder)	

Blend all ingredients and serve on romaine lettuce with sprouts.

VEGETABLE LOAF - 1

20 walnuts-chopped	1/4 cabbage
2 carrots	1 small beet
5 leaves of cilantro	1 garlic clove
1/2 lemon	1/4 cup water
1/4 cup processed vegetables	1 teaspoon coriander
1/2 avocado	1 onion chopped

Place cabbage, carrots and beet into a food processor and process. Blend garlic, lemon, water, coriander, and 1/4 cup of the processed vegetables into a smooth sauce. Add onions and cut up avocado. Make into a small loaf on each plate and serve topped with walnuts and cilantro leaf. This mixture can be put on zucchini crackers. Zucchini can be sliced fresh or dehydrated.

VEGETABLE LOAF - 2

1 cup sunflower seeds - soaked 4 hours or more, then put into a Champion Juicer to grind to a paste

1 cup Romaine Lettuce	1 carrot - grated
4 finely chopped mushrooms	2 teaspoons tamari
3 ribs of celery - finely chopped	1 teaspoon basil

Food process the romaine lettuce and mix all ingredients together and form a loaf. Press down softly in the middle of the loaf to form a canal. Fill with sauce from the following ingredients (Sauce):

1/2 avocado	1 teaspoon tamari

Blend ingredients to a smooth consistency.

CABBAGE TACO

Fill cabbage with shredded carrots, cauliflower, lettuce, mushrooms, cashews, sprouts and broccoli. Put dressing (see salads, dips and dressings) on top.

AVOCADO BOATS

1/4 onion-finely chopped	1 carrot-shredded
1 celery-cut small	1 avocado-halved
Romaine lettuce	

Mix together first three ingredients and place in the middle of each avocado half. Serve on a bed of romaine lettuce. (Can also be made with celery-beet-tomato combination.)

CUCUMBER SHIP

1 rib of celery-cut small	1/2 avocado-smashed
1 branch fresh parsley-cut small	1 teaspoon tamari
1 tomato-cut small	cucumber
salad greens	

Peel cucumber, cut in half lengthwise and hollow out the center. Mix first five ingredients and place mixture into the center of the cucumbers. Place cucumbers on top of greens.

COLORED COLESLAW

1/4 cup walnuts-crush with rolling pin	
1/4 head of white cabbage	1 carrot
1/4 head of purple cabbage	1/4 cup raisins
1/4 cup mayonnaise - see recipe for mayonnaise	

Shred cabbages and carrots, mix with walnuts and raisins and combine with the mayonnaise.

STUFFED RED TOMATO CUPS

2 large ripe tomatoes	1 summer squash-grated
1/2 green pepper-chopped small	2 teaspoons of kelp
1/2 clove garlic	1/4 onion
1/2 avocado-cut small	Salad greens

Cut the top off of the tomato and scoop out the pulp. Mix remaining ingredients with tomato pulp and juice in a bowl. Stuff the tomato and serve on greens.

STUFFED ZUCCHINI

4 mushrooms - cut small	1/2 avocado-cut small
1/4 onion-finely chopped	1 cup corn
1 cup sunflower sprouts - cut small, Mix all vegetables	
1 tablespoon Braggs	1 zucchini

Cut zucchini in half and scoop out seeds. Mix all ingredients except zucchini and place in the middle of zucchini halves.

LEMON CUCUMBER

2 shredded cucumbers	1/4 teaspoon mustard
3 teaspoons flaxseed powder	1/2 lemon
3 teaspoons dill	

Mix all ingredients together and serve in bowls.

Note: Also good with cut up avocado pieces.

CORN CHOWDER

1/2 avocado-cut in small pieces	1 cup raw corn
1/4 onion	1 teaspoon Braggs
5 basil leaves	1 pinch of seaweed
1 squash	1/2 cup water

Place onion, braggs, basil, seaweed, squash and water into blender and blend until smooth. Add corn and avocado and mix all ingredients together. Serve in bowls.

CORN ON THE COB

Avocado	Corn on cob
Sea seasoning	Purple onion - cut small

Take ripe avocado slice and rub onto corn like butter. Sprinkle sea seasoning lightly on corn and roll onto onions.

CORN DELIGHT

1 branch broccoli	1/4 head of cabbage
5 leaves basil	2 cups corn

Food process broccoli, cabbage and basil. Mix together and add corn.

TOBBULEH

1/2 cup chopped fresh parsley	1 tomato-cut small
1 scallion-cut small	1 mint leaf
1 cup bulgur wheat-soaked	Juice of 1/2 lemon
1 tablespoon olive oil	Spices and herbs

Mix the above ingredients and serve.

STUFFED POTATO

1/8 cup onions-finely chopped	2 baked potatoes
1 cup carrot-shredded	1 cup corn
1 celery stick-finely chopped	

Cut potato in half. Scoop out potatoes and mix with vegetables and restuff potatoes. Can add a sauce

TOMATO AND VEGETABLES

5 leaves of red leaf lettuce	1 carrot
1/4 head of purple cabbage	2 tablespoons pine nuts
1 cooked spaghetti squash	

TOMATO SAUCE

Food process the first three ingredients. Place the spaghetti squash on each plate and place the processed vegetables on top. Serve with tomato sauce.

POT LUCK SWEET POTATO PIE

2 large sweet potatoes

Bake sweet potato at low temperature of 250 degrees. Make sure there is no mold on the outside layer of potato. Smash one potato and press onto the bottom of a glass pie pan to form a layer.

Filling:

1/2 avocado	1 carrot-food processed
1 cup fresh peas	1 cup corn
12 leaves of romaine lettuce-cut small	
rib of celery-cut small	

Mix together and put into pie. Use remaining sweet potato to make a layer for the top of the pie.

ASPARAGUS POTATO BOAT

1 potato-scrubbed well and baked   Tomato-cut in pieces
Avocado-cut small   Spinach-cut small
2 asparagus spears-cut small

Cut potato in half and scoop out inside. Mix with tomato, avocado and spinach and asparagus.

JICAMA SANDWICH

2 slices of jicama   1/4 avocado
1 zucchini-shredded   Small piece of onion
Piece of romaine lettuce

Mix the zucchini and onion together. Smash avocado onto jicama and put with the zucchini and onion mixture. Put on lettuce leaf and top with a slice of jicama.

SWEET POTATO SANDWICH

2 thin slices of sweet potato   1 slice of tomato
1/2 avocado-smashed   1 slice onion
1 lettuce leaf

Fill the ingredients between the slices of sweet potato.

LETTUCE SANDWICH

Thick slices of iceberg lettuce   1/2 avocado smashed
1/4 purple onion-finely chopped

Spread a thick layer of avocado onto the iceberg lettuce and sprinkle with onion.

BLT (BROCCOLI, LETTUCE, AND TOMATO)

1 cup cabbage   1 cup broccoli

3 teaspoons powdered coriander seed
1 tablespoon flaxseed oil   1/4 onion
Slices tomato to suit   Lettuce

Bread - life foods or whole grain made without yeast or baking soda. Put first five ingredients into food processor and make mixture into a patty. Prepare the rest of the ingredients and serve on a sandwich.

AVOCADO RYE SANDWICH

1/2 avocado   Rye Bread
1/2 cup sprouts   1 carrot - shredded
2 mushrooms - marinated in tamari sauce
Lettuce

Smash avocado on the bread and fill with the rest of the ingredients.

SPINACH SALAD

30 spinach leaves - food processed
1 carrot - cut up small   1 rib of celery - cut small
1/4 onion - cut small   1/2 cup hummus
2 baked or steamed potatoes - cut up

Mix all ingredients together.

PIZZA
Dough:

2 cups rye or oat flour   1 tablespoon honey
1 tablespoon flaxseed oil
Enough water to get dough consistency

Roll dough in a ball, sprinkle cutting board with flour and roll dough into a large circle. Place into oiled glass pie pan. (Or you may use pita pocket bread as crust)

Sauce:

1/2 cup of tomato sauce   Basil

Put sauce onto dough and bak 300 degrees for 1 hour.

Next layer with vegetables:

1/4 onion   5 leaves spinach
4 mushrooms - sliced   1/2 cup sprouts
1 tomato - sliced

OTHER IDEAS FOR STARCHES BESIDES OATS AND WHEAT:

Millet	Brown Rice
Sweet Potato	Potato
Jerusalem Artichoke	Peas
Corn Noodles	Corn Spaghetti Noodles
Buckwheat Spaghetti Noodles	Carrots
Corn	Spaghetti squash

SALADS

In 1991 I travelled in Europe (Switzerland, Paris and Brussels) and found the salads interesting and different than in the United States.

CARROTS ALA EUROPE

3 carrots   1 lemon

Shred the carrots and place on the middle of plate. Serve with slices of lemon.

SALAD EUROPE

1/2 cup corn   7 leaves of lettuce
1 tomato - sliced

Place the lettuce leaves on the outside of the plate and put the corn and tomato in the middle.

EUROPEAN MIXER

1 tomato - sliced   1/2 cup corn
8 asparagus - cooked   20 string beans - cooked
Plate of lettuce

Place each food in their own section on the plate.

GARBONZO BEAN SALAD

1/2 cup garbonzo beans—soak overnight, sprouted or cooked
1 squash - shredded   Juice of 1 lemon
1 tablespoon flax seed oil   2 teaspoons dill
1 teaspoon herb seasoning   2 teaspoons sorghum
1/4 onion - finely chopped

Mix all ingredients together.

ARTICHOKE SALAD

4 Jerusalem artichokes - cut small   1 carrot - shredded
2 ribs celery - cut small   1/2 turnip - shredded
1/4 onion - cut small   1 tablespoon flax seed oil
3 drops sweetener   10 walnuts - cut small
Juice of 1/2 lemon   Romaine lettuce leaves

Mix all the ingredients and place on the lettuce leaves.

SPROUT SALAD

1/2 avocado	1/4 onion - chopped
1/2 sweet potato - shredded	1/2 squash - shredded
1/2 cup lentil sprouts	1/2 cup pea sprouts
1 tomato	5 spinach leaves

Mix all together and serve with a healthy salad dressing.

COLESLAW

1/2 head of cabbage - grated	1 carrot - grated
1/4 onion - chopped	

Mix above ingredients and serve with dressing.
Dressing:

Juice of 1 lemon	1 teaspoon sea salt
Dulse	Basil
Anise	1/4 cup water

Blend ingredients.

DRESSINGS

LEMON DRESSING

1 avocado - smashed	Juice of 2 lemons
2 teaspoons dill	

Mix all ingredients together.

PINK DRESSING

1/2 beet	1/2 squash
1/4 avocado	Small fresh ginger
1 clove garlic	seaweed
Juice of 1/2 lemon	1/2 cup water
1 tablespoon dill	

Blend all of the ingredients together.

PINEAPPLE DRESSING

Juice of 1 lemon	1/2 cup water
1 tablespoon flax seed powder	1 teaspoon dill
2 dried pineapple rings - cut small	1/8 teaspoon mustard
1 teaspoon honey	1 clove garlic - cut small
Small piece of fresh ginger - finely cut	1 onion - cut small

Mix all ingredients in a bowl.

THOUSAND ISLAND DRESSING

1 tbsp. honey	1 tomato
1 tbsp. Flaxseed	1/2 avocado

Blend all ingredients.

FAVORITE GINGER DRESSING

Small piece of ginger	1 clove garlic
1/4 chopped onion	1 tablespoon flax seed oil
Juice of 1/2 lemon	1/2 avocado
1/2 cup water	

Blend all ingredients together. Add finely cut garlic and onion.

TOMATO DRESSING

2 tomatoes	1 clove garlic - cut small
1 tablespoon flax seed powder	1 teaspoon dill

Blend all ingredients together.

SESAME DILL DRESSING

2 tablespoons sesame seed powder	
2 teaspoons dill	1/4 cup olive oil
Pinch of sea salt	Juice of 2 small lemons
1/2 cup avocado	1 rib celery - cut small
1/2 cup water	1/4 squash - cut small

Blend all together.

HUMMUS DRESSING

1/2 cup hummus bean dip powder (Casbah or sprouted chick peas)	
1/2 carrot -cut small	1 tablespoon olive oil
Juice of 1 lemon	2 teaspoons dill
1/2 cup water	

Blend all ingredients together.

HOLIDAY CRANBERRY SAUCE

1/4 bag cranberries	2 oranges - peeled
1/2 cup honey or sweetener	
1 bottle of all fruit natural cranberry sauce by K.W. Knudes	

Food process all of the ingredients.

MAYONNAISE

1 cup cashews
1/4 cup cauliflower
Juice of 1 lemon
1 tablespoon honey

1/4 cup safflower oil
1/2 cup water
1 teaspoon mustard

Food process the cashews and cauliflower and add the water. Slowly add the oil until thick and place the rest of the ingredients into a blender and blend until smooth. The mixture will be thick.

CASHEW MAYONNAISE

1 cup cashews
lemon juice

2 tablespoons honey
1/2 cup water

Blend until creamy.

APPETIZERS

CELERY STICKS

1 avocado - smashed
1 green pepper - cut small

1 onion - cut small
Celery sticks

Mix the first three ingredients and spread in the middle of the celery sticks.

PIZZA QUAKERS

Rye seed (ground in coffee grinder)
Broccoli
Tomatoes
Tomato paste - heated

Basil
Zucchini or rice crackers

Food process the broccoli, rye, basil and tomato. Spread the heated tomato paste onto the crackers, then top with broccoli mixture.

STUFFED MUSHROOMS

1 carrot
1/2 cup corn
1/2 avocado
1/2 cup sprouts - cut small
Large mushroom caps

1 rib celery
1/4 onion
1/4 cup water
1/4 cup pine nuts

Food process the first six ingredients and mix with the sprouts and pine nuts. Stuff the mushrooms with the mixture.

POTATO AND ZUCCHINI

1 zucchini - sliced   1 cup mashed potatoes
1 tomato - sliced

Spread the mashed potatoes on the zucchini slice and top with a
slice of tomato.

FINGER FOODS

I personally like picking up my food with my hands. This
gives me a more natural feeling.

Here are some of my favorite foods to use with dips.

Broccoli   Cabbage
Romaine lettuce   Carrots
Celery   Squash
Turnip   Cauliflower
Beets
Jerusalem artichokes

DIPS

BEET DIP

1/2 beet - cut very small   1/2 avocado - smashed
2 teaspoons cinnamon

Blend all ingredients together.

HERB DIP

1 avocado - smashed   1 tablespoon braggs
1 teaspoon Italian seasoning   2 teaspoons basil
1 teaspoon seaweed

Blend all of the above ingredients together.

HUMMUS DIP

1 cup of garbanzo beans, soaked over night
1/2 cup ground sesame seeds   1 large clove of garlic
1/2 cup olive oil - cold pressed 1 lemon
1/2 cup water to blend

Blend in a blender until a thick consistency. For more spice, add
more garlic and herbs or 2 teaspoons of curry powder.

CARROT DIP

1 carrot - cut very small   1/2 avocado - smashed
1 tablespoon Braggs

Blend all of the above ingredients.

AVOCADO DIP

1 smashed avocado   1/4 onion - finely chopped
1 clove garlic - finely chopped   Juice of 1/2 lemon
Tomato - finely chopped   Cilantro

Mix all of the above ingredients.

CORN DIP

1 ear of corn - cut off the cob   1 avocado - smashed
Mix the above ingredients.

GINGER DIP

1 avocado   1 small piece ginger
2 teaspoons dill

Blend the above ingredients.

POTATO GARLIC DIP

1 baked potato   2 cloves garlic - finely cut
1/4 avocado - smashed

Blend all of the above ingredients.

BEVERAGES

CALLI BEVERAGE-Sunrider International
FORTUNE DELIGHT-Sunrider International
HERBAL DRINKS-health food stores
SWEETNER can be substituted for 2 tablespoons
    of maple syrup or honey

LEMONADE

1/2 lemon - squeezed   10 drops sweetener
1-1/2 cups water

Mix all together.

LEMON ORANGEADE

2 fresh lemons - squeezed   2 oranges - squeezed
10 drops sweetener - optional   3 cups water
Mix all together.

GINGERADE

1 small piece of ginger   1 lemon - squeezed
3 tbsp. honey or maple syrup   3 cups of water

Mix all together.

ALMOND MILK

20 almonds-soaked overnight and then peeled
20 drops of sweetener   2 cups of water

Blend together; afterwards, put through screen to get out nut pieces.

ASSIMILAID NUT MILK

5 Assimilaid capsules
10 drops sweetner   10 pecans
2 cups water

Blend all ingredients together and then put through a screen to separate the nuts from the milk.

ALMOND CINNAMON MILK

1 teaspoon cinnamon   1 teaspoon nutmeg
20 drops sweetener, molasses or maple syrup
2 cups of water   20 almonds

Blend all ingredients together and then put through a screen to separate the nuts from the milk.

PECAN MILK

20 Pecans   20 drops sweetener
2 cups of water

Blend all ingredients until the nuts are well incorporated.

CINNAMON DELIGHT SHAKE

8 dates   2 teaspoons cinnamon
1 tablespoon flaxseed powder   1/2 carrot
10 drops sweetener   1/4 avocado
4 cups water

Food process all ingredients and blend.

DATE BANANA SHAKE

8 dates fresh or soaked   1 Banana
3 cups water

Blend all ingredients.

PINA BANANA

1/4 fresh pineapple   1 banana
1 tablespoon coconut shredded 2 dates
2 cups water

Blend all ingredients.

CHOCOLATE SHAKE

2 tablespoons chocolate powder 10 drops sweetener
1/4 cup nuplus plain   1 cup of water

Blend.

CAROB MILK

2 tablespoon nuplus simply herbs-Sunrider International
1 cup of water   2 tablespoon carob
10 drops of sweetener

Blend.

WATERMELON JUICE

Take the seeds out of the watermelon and put watermelon through a juicer or blender. The rind of an organic watermelon can also be used.

FRESH ORANGE JUICE

Put fresh oranges through a juicer and serve.

FRESH APPLE JUICE

Put apples through juicer.

CARROT JUICE

Put carrots through juicer and serve. (I personally like my carrots peeled then put through juicer.)

BEET CELERY CARROT JUICE

1 beet   2 carrots
1 rib of celery

Put vegetables through a juicer and serve.

DESERTS

BANANA ICE CREAM

5 frozen bananas

Take 5 fresh bananas and put in plastic Zip Lock bag. Freeze overnight and put through Champion Juicer.

FRUITY ICE CREAM

Frozen bananas   1 peach
4 strawberries

Put into a Champion juicer with a blank inside.

FRESH FIG ICE CREAM

10 fresh figs   4 frozen bananas
3 dates

Put through a Champion juicer using the blank.

FIG ICE CREAM

10 figs dried-soaked overnight   1/4 cup water
10 almonds-soaked and peeled   1 teaspoon vanilla
1/4 cup maple syrup

Blend ingredients and then put into small bowls and freeze.

STRAWBERRY ICE CREAM

7 frozen strawberries   2 frozen bananas

Put strawberries and bananas through a Champion Juicer.

CAROB ICE CREAM

5 bananas   1/2 cup carob powder
pecans - cut small

Smash bananas in bowl, add the carob and nuts and freeze.

MINT ICE CREAM

1 avocado   1/4 cup honey
20 pecans   1/4 cup water
1 teaspoon peppermint

Blend first four ingredients in a blender reserving 2 pecans. Put in 2 small bowls and sprinkle with mint and place a pecan on top. Freeze until hard about 3 hours.

BANANA SPLIT

1 fresh banana   2 frozen bananas

Put bananas through the Champion Juicer then make the following sauce.

Sauce:

1/4 cup carob or chocolate   1/4 cup of nuplus
20 drops sweetener   1/2 cup water
10 walnuts-crushed with a rolling pin

Blend nuplus, carob, sweetener and water (or carob and honey). Add the sauce to the bananas and sprinkle with nuts.

AVOCADO ICE CREAM

3 tablespoons honey   1 avocado
1/2 cup water

Blend avocado, water and honey together and freeze in small cups. For avocado butter ice cream just add 2 tablespoons of peanut butter.

DATE CAKE

1 cup walnuts   1 carrot
3 dates   1/4 cup coconut
8 dates

Food process first four ingredients and place half of the mixture in an oblong shape. Food process the 8 dates and place on top of the walnut mixture. Place the remaining walnut mixture on top of the dates.

APPLE CAKE

1/4 cup coconut   1 cup walnuts
1 carrot   2 dates
20 raisins   1 apple
1/2 cup raisins

Frosting:

2 apples   3 dates

Food process the first group of ingredients. Stir the mixture and raisins together and form a thick high oblong shape. Food process the remaining apples and dates and frost the cake.

DATE PUDDING

1/4 cup Nuplus   1/4 cup water
5 drops sweetener   5 dates

Blend all ingredients until thick.

CORN PUDDING

1 ear of corn - cut off the cob   1/2 avocado
2 teaspoons cinnamon   10 drops sweetener
2 teaspoons nutmeg

Blend all of the ingredients.

BANANA PUDDING

Put fresh bananas through Champion juicer.

FAST RICE PUDDING

1 cup brown rice - cooked   1 teaspoon cinnamon
1 tablespoon honey   1/4 cup raisins

Mix all of the ingredients together.

RICE PUDDING #2

1 apple   1/2 celery
1/2 carrot   1/4 cup water
1 cup rice   1 tablespoon honey
1 teaspoon cinnmon

Blend the above ingredients with:

1 cup rice - cooked   1/4 cup raisins

Stir mixtures together and sprinkle top of pudding with Sunrider's Vitadophalus.

PUMPKIN PUDDING

1 cup of raw or cooked pumpkin   1 tablespoon honey
1/4 cup water   1/4 cup raisins
shredded carrots
Cashew Whipped Cream (see following recipe)

Mix the first three ingredients in a blender and serve in small cups with raisins. Top with shredded carrots and a dollop of cashew whipped cream.

CASHEW WHIPPED CREAM

1 cup cashews   1/4 cauliflower
1/2 teaspoon vanilla extract   1/2 cup water
2 tablespoons honey *or* 4 tablespoons maple syrup

Blend to a thick texture.

CARROT DESSERT

2 rings of dried pineapple - cut small   1 carrot shredded
4 dates - cut small

Mix all of the ingredients together.

APPLE RAISIN

1 cup apple sauce (apples blended)
1/4 cup raisins   1 celery - cut small
1 apple - cut small   1/4 cup raisins

Food process the apple sauce and raisins until creams. Stir the apple sauce mixture together with the remaining ingredients.

HONEY YAM

1 yam or sweet potato - cooked   1 tablespoon honey
20 raisins   Cinnamon

Peel off potato skin and press the raisins onto the yam. Pour on honey and sprinkle with cinnamon.

PUMPKIN PIE

Crust:

2 cups walnuts   1 cup carrots

Food process ingredients and line a glass pie pan.
Filling:

1 cup raw pumpkin   1/2 avocado
1 teaspoon cinnamon   1 teaspoon nutmeg
1/4 cup maple syrup

Combine the filling ingredients and blend until thick and creamy. Fill the pie crust.

APPLE PIE

Crust:

1 cup walnuts   1 large carrot
4 dates   1/2 apple
raisins

Blend the first four ingredients in a food processor and line a glass pie pan with mixture. Press raisins into mixture.

Filling:

5 red apples   1 teaspoon cinnamon
1 tablespoon flax seed powder   1/4 cup raisins
1/4 cup water   2 green apples shredded

Blend the filling ingredients then mix with the shredded apples. Fill the pie shell.

DEBBIE'S FRUIT SALAD

1 cup blueberries   6 strawberries - sliced
3 peaches - cut up   1/2 pineapple - cut up
2 cups grapes

Mix all the ingredients together.

MELON SALAD

1/2 watermelon   1 cantalope
1 honeydew

Cut fruit into bite size pieces, mix and serve.

ALL AMERICAN FRUIT SALAD

3 bananas - (slice just before serving)
4 oranges - cut up   4 apples - cut up
2 cups grapes

Mix all ingredients together.

NATURE'S CANDY

DATE PECAN BALLS

20 dates   1/4 cup pecans
2 tablespoons of shredded coconut   1/2 cup raisins

Food process the first three ingredients, form into balls and roll in coconut.

DATE COCONUT CANDY

10 dates   2 tablespoons coconut
Pecans

Food process the ingredients, roll into balls and press a pecan on top of each one.

MARBLED CAROB HALAVEH BALLS

1/2 cup sesame seed powder-ground in grinder or coffee mill
3 tablespoons carob powder   1/4 cup honey hard

Mix sesame and honey together. Then mix carob powder and sesame honey mixture together and make a swirl or marble effect. Form balls or press into a small flat square pan. You can also make a sauce out of the carob honey mixture and place on top of halaveh.

DATE PECAN

4 dates   4 pecans

Open up dates, take seed out and replace with pecan. Close date around pecan.

CAROB ROLL

1 cup pecans or walnuts   1/2 cup raisins
1/2 cup dates   1/4 cup carob powder

Food process the raisins, pecans or walnuts and dates. Make a roll and refrigerate. Slice the next day. Dust with carob powder.

HEALTH COOKIES

1 ounce wheat grass juice   1 carrot
2 tablespoons flax seed   1 cup walnuts
1 cup raisins   1 capsule ginseng
1 cup sprouts   Carob powder
2 tablespoons honey or other sweetener

Grind the above ingredients together and make into balls. Flatten with spoon and dust with carob powder.

FIG COOKIES

4 figs   20 dates
1 tablespoon flax seed powder   30 pecans
1 carrot   1 capsule ginseng

Food process the figs and dates together. Make a cookie base from the pecans, flax seed powder, carrot and ginseng by processing together. Spoon the fig and date mixture into the middle of the cookie base mixture.

ANN WIGMORE SPECIAL BANANA SUNFLOWER COOKIES

1 cup sunflower seeds   2 bananas

Blend ingredients in blender and spoon onto dehydrator sheets. Dehydrate for 2 days. Flip if not drying fast enough.

DATE WALNUT COOKIES

2 cups walnuts - food processed   1 carrot - food processed
2 dates - food processed   1 teaspoon cinnamon
1 teaspoon cloves   1 teaspoon vanilla
1/4 cup honey   8 dates - cut up

Mix all ingredients together and add cut up dates. Dehydrate or put in oven at 175° degrees for 3 hours - flip over after 1 1/2 hours.

GINGER SNAPS

Small piece of fresh ginger   1 teaspoon cinnamon
1/4 cup oats   1/4 cup buckwheat
2 teaspoons flax seed   20 drops sweetener
2 tablespoons molasses   2 tablespoons sorgham
1/2 cup water

Mix ingredients together, shape into cookies and put in dehydrator overnight or bake at 275° for about 20 min.

ROCKY ROAD CAROB COOKIES

1/4 cup carob   1/4 cup oats
1/4 cup buckwheat   2 tablespoons molasses
10 drops sweetener   2 tablespoons sorgham
1 tablespoon flax seed oil   1/2 cup water
1 smashed banana   6 walnuts - cut up
1/4 cup raisins   2 dates - cut up

Mix all ingredients together, shape into cookies and dehydrate overnight or bake at 275° for about 20 min.

SESAME COOKIES

3/4 cup sesame seeds- ground in a coffee grinder
1 cup buckwheat   4 large dates
1/4 cup pecans - chopped up   1/4 cup raisins
1/4 cup honey   1 teaspoon vanilla
1 teaspoon cinnamon   1 teaspoon nutmeg
1 cup water - add until right consistency

Mix all ingredients together, shape into cookies and dehydrate or bake for 45 minutes at 250° degrees.

PRODUCTS USED

Champion Juicer - Plastaket Mfg. Co. Inc., Lodi, California -used for ice cream, juice, nut butter.

Food Processor - sauces, grating.

Blender - sauces, salad dressings, soup, nut milks. I used the Osterizer Blender which has an attachment for a small food processor.

Coffee Mill (Krups) - grinds seeds and nuts to a flour.

Hand Food Grater - grates carrots.

Metal Meat grinder - grinds nuts, vegetables, dried fruits.

Sunrider whole food herbs - Beauty Pearl, Quinary, NuPlus, Calli, Fortune Delight, Top, Ese. (1-800-448-8786)

Par de Arco - medicinal herb used only for a short time.

Acidopholous - Sunrider's Vitadolphalus Twin Labs Allerdolpalus. (The Staff of Life L-Salvarius - 1-509-738-2345)

Flaxseed Oil - use for salad dressings, lotions for face, soups, hands and hair.

Fresh wheat grass juice

Yeast free bread - Pacific Bakery, 514 S. Hill Street,

PO Box 950, Oceanside,Ca 92049, Ph No (619)-757-6020

Buy herbs from the health food store because this will give you the best chance to get them free of irradiation.

-allspice	-almonds
-basil	-brazil nuts
-caraway seed powdered	-carob
-cashews	-celery seed
-cinnamon	-dates
-dill	-dulse powder or pieces
-flaxseed powder	-garlic
-ginger	-Italian seasoning
-licorice	-mustard seed powder
-nutmeg	-olive oil
-onion	-oregano
-pecans	-poppy seed
-pumpkin seeds	-raisins
-rosemary	-sesame seed and powdered
-sunflower seeds	-tamari or Braggs
-thyme	-vanilla
-walnuts	

TABLE OF FOOD COMPOSITION

FRUITS	Measure	Weight g	Calories	Protein g	Fats g	Carbohydrates g	Calcium mg	Iron mg	Magnesium mg
Apples, raw, whole	1 med	130	76	0.3	0.8	17.0	9.0	0.39	10.4
Apricots, raw	1 med	38	19	0.4	0.1	4.1	6.5	0.19	4.6
Avocado	1 lg	216	361	4.5	33.0	12.0	22.0	1.30	97.0
Banana, raw	1 med	150	128	1.6	0.3	30.0	12.0	1.10	49.5
Blackberries, raw	1 cup	144	84	1.7	1.3	17.0	46.0	1.30	45.0
Blueberries, raw	1 cup	140	87	1.0	0.7	19.0	21.0	1.40	8.4
Cantaloupe, raw	¼	100	30	0.7	0.1	7.5	14.0	0.40	16.0
Cherries, sour, raw	1 cup	200	116	2.4	0.6	28.6	44.0	0.80	28.0
Cherries, sweet, raw	1 cup	200	140	2.6	0.6	32.0	44.0	0.80	22.5
Cranberries, raw	1 cup	100	460	0.4	0.7	10.8	14.0	0.50	-
Dates, dried	1 med	10	27	0.2	t	6.3	5.9	0.30	5.8
Elderberries, raw	1 cup	457	329	11.9	2.3	75.0	174.0	7.30	-
Figs, dried	1 lg	21	58	0.9	0.3	13.0	26.0	0.63	14.9
Figs, raw	1 med	38	30	0.5	0.1	6.8	13.0	0.23	7.6
Gooseberries	1 cup	150	59	1.2	0.3	14.6	27.0	0.75	13.5
Grapefruit, raw, red flesh, 5″ diam.	1 med	260	108	1.3	0.3	25.0	46.0	1.14	31.2
Grapes, American Concord	1 cup	153	106	2.0	1.5	21.0	24.0	0.61	19.9
Grapes, European, Muscat, or Tokay	1 cup	160	107	1.0	0.5	25.0	19.0	0.64	9.6
Grapes, green, seedless	1 cup	200	102	1.0	0.2	27.2	16.0	0.60	-

Phosphorus mg	Potassium mg	Sodium mg	Vitamin A IU	(Thiamine) B$_1$ mg	(Riboflavin) B$_2$ mg	Vitamin B$_6$ mg	Vitamin B$_{12}$ mcg	Folic Acid mg	Niacin mg	Vitamin C mg	Vitamin E mg
13.0	143	1.0	117	0.040	0.03	0.039	0	0.003	0.13	5.20	0.40
8.7	107	0.4	1,026	0.010	0.02	0.023	0	0.001	0.23	0.38	-
91.0	1,305	8.6	626	0.240	0.43	0.907	0	0.060	3.46	31.00	-
39.0	555	1.5	285	0.080	0.09	0.765	0	0.010	1.05	15.00	0.33
27.0	245	1.4	288	0.040	0.06	0.075	0	0.021	0.60	30.00	-
18.0	113	1.0	140	0.040	0.08	0.094	0	0.011	0.70	20.00	-
16.0	251	12.0	3,400	0.040	0.03	0.086	0	0.007	0.60	33.00	0.14
38.0	218	4.0	2,000	0.100	0.12	0.170	-	0.012	0.80	20.00	-
38.0	382	4.0	220	0.100	0.12	0.064	0	0.012	0.80	20.00	-
10.0	2	82.0	40	0.030	0.02	0.040	-	-	0.10	11.00	-
6.3	65	0.1	5	0.016	0.01	0.015	0	-	0.20	0	-
127.0	1,371	-	2,742	0.320	0.27	-	-	-	2.29	-	-
16.0	134	7.1	17	0.020	0.02	0.037	0	0.007	0.15	0	-
8.4	74	0.8	30	0.020	0.02	0.043	0	0.010	0.15	0.76	-
22.5	233	1.5	435	-	-	-	-	-	-	49.50	-
46.0	385	2.9	1,144	0.160	0.06	0.090	0	0.010	0.57	105.00	0.58
18.0	242	4.6	153	0.080	0.05	0.120	0	0.010	0.46	6.12	-
32.0	277	4.8	160	0.080	0.05	-	-	-	0.48	6.40	-
26.0	220	8.0	140	0.080	0.02	-	-	-	0.40	4.0	-

TABLE OF FOOD COMPOSITION

FRUITS	Measure	Weight g	Calories	Protein g	Fats g	Carbohydrates g	Calcium mg	Iron mg	Magnesium mg
Lemon juice, fresh	1 T	15	4	0.1	t	1.2	1.0	0.03	4.5
Nectarine, raw	1 med	87	50	0.5	t	12.0	3.1	0.39	11.3
Olive, green, pickled	1 lg	7	9	0.1	0.9	0.1	4.3	0.11	1.54
Olive, ripe, canned	1 lg	7	13	0.1	1.4	0.2	7.4	0.12	-
Orange, fresh	1 med	180	88	1.8	0.4	20.0	74.0	0.72	19.8
Papaya, raw	1 lg	400	156	2.4	0.4	40.0	80.0	1.20	-
Peach, fresh	1 med	114	43	0.7	0.1	10.0	10.0	0.57	11.4
Pears, fresh	1 med	182	111	1.3	0.7	27.8	15.0	0.60	12.7
Persimmon, Japanese, raw	1 med	125	96	0.9	0.5	22.0	7.5	0.38	10.0
Pineapple, raw	1 cup	140	73	0.5	0.3	17.0	24.0	0.70	17.0
Plum, fresh, 2" Damson	1 med	60	29	0.3	t	6.7	7.2	0.30	5.4
Prunes, dried, raw	1 lg	10	26	0.2	0.1	6.2	5.1	0.39	0.4
Raisins, dried	1 cup	160	462	4.0	0.3	111.0	99.0	5.60	56.0
Raspberries, red, raw	1 cup	133	76	1.6	0.7	16.0	29.0	1.20	26.6
Strawberries, raw	1 cup	149	55	1.0	0.7	11.0	31.0	1.49	17.9
Tangerine, raw	1 lg	114	52	0.9	0.2	12.0	46.0	0.46	-
Watermelon, 4" x 8" piece	1 wedge	925	241	4.6	1.8	52.0	65.0	4.63	84.2

Phosphorus mg	Potassium mg	Sodium mg	Vitamin A IU	(Thiamine) B$_1$ mg	(Riboflavin) B$_2$ mg	Vitamin B$_6$ mg	Vitamin B$_{12}$ mcg	Folic Acid mg	Niacin mg	Vitamin C mg	Vitamin E mg
2.0	85	0.1	3	0.010	t	0.030	-	t	0.01	7.00	-
19.0	229	4.7	1,287	t	t	0.015	0	0.017	-	10.00	-
1.2	4	168.0	21	0	0	-	0	-	-	t	-
1.2	2	53.0	4.9	t	t	0.001	0	t	-	-	-
36.0	360	1.8	360	0.180	0.05	0.108	0	0.010	0.72	90.00	0.43
64.0	936	12.0	7,000	0.160	0.16	-	0	-	1.20	224.00	-
22.0	234	1.1	1,516	0.020	0.06	0.027	0	0.004	1.14	7.98	-
20.0	237	3.6	36	0.040	0.08	0.034	0	-	0.18	7.28	-
33.0	218	7.5	3,388	0.040	0.03	-	-	-	0.13	13.80	-
11.0	204	1.4	98	1.300	0.04	0.120	0	0.008	0.28	24.00	-
11.0	102	0.6	150	0.040	0.02	0.030	0	-	0.30	3.60	-
7.9	69	0.8	160	0.010	0.02	0.020	0	0.001	0.16	0.30	-
162.0	1,221	43.0	32	0.180	0.13	0.380	0	0.020	0.80	1.60	-
29.0	223	1.3	173	0.040	0.12	0.080	0	0.007	1.20	33.00	-
31.0	244	1.5	89	0.050	0.10	0.080	0	0.013	0.89	88.00	0.19
21.0	144	2.3	479	0.070	0.02	0.076	0	0.008	0.11	35.00	-
93.0	925	9.2	5,458	0.280	0.28	0.630	0	0.009	1.85	65.00	

TABLE OF FOOD COMPOSITION

NUTS, NUT PRODUCTS, AND SEEDS	Measure	Weight g	Calories	Protein g	Fats g	Carbohydrates g	Calcium mg	Iron mg	Magnesium mg
Almonds, dried	1 cup	140	765	26.0	76.0	26.0	328.0	6.58	378.0
Brazil nuts, unsalted	1 cup	300	1,962	42.0	201.0	32.7	558.0	10.00	675.0
Butternuts	5 avg	15	96	3.6	9.2	1.3	-	1.00	-
Cashews, unsalted	1 cup	100	569	15.0	45.0	26.0	39.0	3.80	274.0
Chestnuts, fresh	1 cup	200	382	5.8	3.0	84.2	54.0	3.40	82.0
Coconut, fresh	1 cup	100	346	3.5	35.3	9.4	13.0	1.70	46.0
Hazelnuts (filberts)	11 avg	15	97	1.6	9.5	3.0	38.0	0.50	27.6
Hickory nuts	15 sm	15	101	2.1	10.1	2.0	-	0.40	24.0
Peanuts, roasted, w/skin	1 cup	240	1,397	60.0	107.0	48.0	173.0	5.28	420.0
Pistachio nuts	1 cup	100	594	19.0	54.0	19.0	131.0	7.30	158.0
Pumpkin and Squash kernels	1 cup	230	1,271	67.0	107.0	35.0	117.0	26.00	-
Sesame seeds, dry, decorticated	1 cup	230	1,339	42.0	123.0	41.0	253.0	5.50	416.0
Sunflower seeds, dry	1 cup	100	560	24.0	43.0	19.0	120.0	7.10	38.0
Walnuts, Black	1 cup	100	628	21.0	59.6	15.1	t	6.00	190.0
Walnuts, English, raw	1 cup	100	651	15.0	59.0	15.0	99.0	3.10	131.0

Phosphorus mg	Potassium mg	Sodium mg	Vitamin A IU	(Thiamine) B_1 mg	(Riboflavin) B_2 mg	Vitamin B_6 mg	Vitamin B_{12} mcg	Folic Acid mg	Niacin mg	Vitamin C mg	Vitamin E mg
706.0	1,082	5.6	0	0.340	1.29	0.140	0	0.063	4.90	t	-
2,088.0	2,145	3.0	t	3.300	0.36	0.510	0	0.015	4.60	30.00	-
373.0	464	15.0	100	0.430	0.25	-	0	-	1.80	-	-
176.0	908	12.0	-	0.440	0.44	-	-	-	0.12	-	-
95.0	256	23.0	0	0.050	0.02	0.044	0	0.028	0.50	3.00	-
48.0	71	0.1	16	0.069	0.08	-	-	0.010	0.80	1.10	-
54.0	-	-	-	0.080	-	-	-	-	0	-	-
976.0	1,683	12.0	t	0.770	0.32	0.700	0	0.140	40.00	2.40	18.50
500.0	972	-	230	0.670	-	-	-	-	1.40	0	-
2,631.0	-	-	161	0.550	0.44	-	-	5.50	-	-	-
1,361.0	-	-	-	0.410	0.30	-	-	-	12.40	0	-
837.0	920	30.0	50	1.960	0.23	-	-	-	5.40	-	-
570.0	460	3.0	300	0.220	0.11	-	-	0.077	0.70	-	-
380.0	450	2.0	30	0.330	0.13	0.730	0	0.080	0.90	2	

TABLE OF FOOD COMPOSITION

VEGETABLES	Measure	Weight g	Calories	Protein g	Fats g	Carbohydrates g	Calcium mg	Iron mg	Magnesium mg
Artichoke, raw	1 sm	100	44	2.9	0.2	10.6	51.0	1.30	-
Asparagus, raw	1 spear	16	4	0.4	t	0.8	3.5	1.60	-
Beans, green, cooked	1 cup	125	31	2.0	0.2	8.9	62.5	.75	40.0
Beans, Lima, green, raw	1 cup	160	197	13.0	0.8	35.4	83.2	4.50	10.7
Bean sproutes (mung beans) raw	1 cup	50	-	1.9	0.1	3.3	10.0	0.65	-
Cabbage, shredded, raw	1 cup	105	25	1.4	0.2	5.7	51.5	0.42	14.0
Cabbage, red, raw	1 cup	100	31	2.0	0.2	6.9	42.0	0.80	35.0
Carrots, sliced, raw	1 lg	100	42	1.1	0.2	9.7	37.0	0.70	23.0
Cauliflower, raw	1 cup	100	27	2.7	0.2	5.2	25.0	1.10	24.0
Celery, stalk, raw	1 lg	50	8	0.4	t	2.0	0.2	0.15	11.0
Chickpeas (garbanzos), dry, raw	½ cup	100	360	20.5	4.8	61.0	150.0	6.90	-
Chives, chopped, raw	1 T	10	3	0.2	t	0.6	7.0	0.20	-
Corn, on-the-cob, raw	1 ear	100	96	3.5	1.0	22.0	3.0	0.70	48.0
Cucumber, raw, not pared	½ med	50	8	0.5	t	1.7	13.0	0.60	6.0
Endive (escarole) raw	1 cup	228	46	3.9	0.2	9.3	17.8	39.00	22.8
Garlic	1 bulb	2	2	0.1	t	0.6	0.6	0.03	-
Kohlrabi, raw, sliced	1 cup	140	41	2.8	0.1	9.2	57.0	0.70	52.0
Leeks, raw	1 cup	200	104	4.4	0.6	22.4	104.0	2.20	46.0
Lettuce, Bibb, Boston	3½ oz	100	14	1.2	0.2	2.5	35.0	2.00	-
Lettuce, Iceberg (head)	3½ oz	100	13	0.9	0.1	2.9	20.0	0.50	11.0

Phosphorus mg	Potassium mg	Sodium mg	Vitamin A IU	(Thiamine) B$_1$ mg	(Riboflavin) B$_2$ mg	Vitamin B$_6$ mg	Vitamin B$_{12}$ mcg	Folic Acid mg	Niacin mg	Vitamin C mg	Vitamin E mg
88.0	430	43.0	160	0.080	0.05	-	-	-	1.00	12.00	-
9.9	44	0.3	144	0.030	0.03	0.020	-	0.020	0.24	5.30	-
46.3	189	5.0	675	0.090	0.11	0.100	0	0.040	0.75	15.00	-
227.0	1,040	3.2	46.4	0.380	0.19	0.270	-	0.050	2.24	46.40	-
32.0	112	2.5	10	0.070	0.07	-	-	-	0.40	10.00	-
31.5	245	21.0	137	0.050	0.05	0.170	0	0.034	0.32	44.00	-
-	268	26.0	40	0.090	0.06	-	-	-	0.40	61.00	-
36.0	341	47.0	11,000	0.060	0.05	0.150	0	0.008	0.60	8.00	0.11
56.0	295	13.0	60	0.110	0.11	0.210	0	0.022	0.70	78.00	-
14.0	171	63.0	120	0.020	0.02	0.030	0	0.004	0.15	4.50	0.19
331.0	797	26.0	50	0.310	0.15	0.54	-	0.130	2.00	-	-
4.0	25	-	580	0.080	0.13	-	-	-	0.10	6.00	-
111.0	280	-	400	.15	0.12	-	-	-	1.70	12.00	-
14.0	80	3.0	125	0.015	0.02	0.021	0	0.004	0.10	5.50	-
123.0	6,826	31.9	7,524	0.160	0.32	0.050	0	0.107	1.14	22.80	-
4.0	11	0.4	t	0.010	t	-	-	-	0.01	0.30	-
71.0	521	11.2	28	0.080	0.06	-	-	-	0.42	92.00	-
100.0	694	10.0	80	0.220	0.12	-	-	-	1.00	34.00	3.80
26.0	264	9.0	970	0.060	0.06	-	-	-	0.03	8.00	-
22.0	175	9.0	330	0.060	0.06	0.055	0	0.021	0.30	6.00	0.06

TABLE OF FOOD COMPOSITION

VEGETABLES	Measure	Weight g	Calories	Protein g	Fats g	Carbohydrates g	Calcium mg	Iron mg	Magnesium mg
Lettuce, leaf	3½ oz	100	18	1.3	0.3	3.5	68.0	1.40	-
Lettuce, Romaine	3½ oz	100	18	1.3	0.3	3.5	68.0	1.40	11.0
Onions, green, raw	1 bulb	8	4	0.1	t	0.8	3.2	0.05	-
Parsley, chopped, raw	1 cup	56	25	2.0	0.3	4.8	114.0	3.50	23.0
Peppers, sweet, green, raw	1 lg	100	22	1.2	0.2	4.8	9.0	0.70	18.0
Potato, baked, w/skin	1 med	100	93	2.6	0.1	21.1	9.0	0.70	22.0
Pumpkin, raw	½ cup	100	26	1.0	0.1	6.5	21.0	8.00	12.0
Radish, raw, red	1 sm	10	2	0.1	t	0.4	3.0	0.10	1.5
Rutabagas, raw	1 cup	150	69	1.6	1.5	16.5	99.0	0.60	22.5
Spinach, raw	1 cup	100	26	3.2	0.3	4.3	93	3.10	88.0
Squash, summer, raw	1 cup	200	38	2.2	0.2	8.4	56.0	0.80	32.0
Squash, winter, boiled, mashed	1 cup	200	76	2.2	0.6	18.4	40.0	1.00	34.0
Sweet potato, baked	1 sm	100	141	2.1	0.5	32.5	40.0	0.90	31.0
Tomato, raw	1 med	150	33	1.6	0.3	7.1	19.5	0.75	21.0
Turnip, raw	½ cup	100	30	1.0	0.2	6.6	39.0	0.50	20.0
Turnip, tops, raw	1 cup	100	28	3.0	0.3	5.0	246.0	1.80	58.0
Water chestnuts, Chinese, raw	4 avg	25	20	0.3	t	4.7	1.0	0.15	-
Watercress	1 cup	50	10	1.1	0.1	1.5	75.5	0.85	10.0

Phosphorus mg	Potassium mg	Sodium mg	Vitamin A IU	(Thiamine) B_1 mg	(Riboflavin) B_2 mg	Vitamin B_6 mg	Vitamin B_{12} mcg	Folic Acid mg	Niacin mg	Vitamin C mg	Vitamin E mg
25.0	264	9.0	1,900	0.050	0.08	-	-	0.044	0.40	18.00	-
25.0	264	9.0	1,900	0.050	0.08	-	-	-	0.40	18.00	-
3.1	18	0.4	t	0.004	t	-	0	0.001	0.03	2.00	-
35.3	407	25.0	4,760	0.070	0.11	0.090	0	0.020	0.67	96.30	3.10
22.0	213	13.0	420	0.080	0.08	0.260	0	0.007	0.50	128.00	-
65.0	503	4.0	t	0.100	0.04	0.233	-	-	1.70	20.00	0.03
44.0	340	1.0	1,600	0.050	0.11	-	-	-	0.60	9.00	
3.1	32	1.8	1	0.003	t	t	0	0.001	0.03	2.60	-
58.5	360	7.5	870	0.110	0.11	-	-	-	1.60	64.30	-
51.0	470	71.0	8,100	0.100	0.20	-	-	-	0.60	51.00	-
58.0	404	2.0	820	0.100	0.18	0.126	-	0.034	2.00	44.00	-
64.0	516	2.0	7,000	0.080	0.20	0.182	0	0.024	0.80	16.00	-
58.0	300	12.0	8,100	0.090	0.07	0.218	0	0.015	0.70	22.00	-
40.5	366	1.5	1,390	0.090	0.06	0.150	0	0.012	1.95	34.50	0.60
30.0	268	49.0	-	0.040	0.07	-	-	-	0.60	36.00	-
58.0	312	-	7,600	0.210	0.39	-	-	-	0.80	139.00	-
16.3	125	5.0	0	0.040	0.05	-	-	-	0.25	1.00	-
27.0	141	21.0	2,450	0.040	0.08	-	-	-	0.45	39.50	

Appendix 3

RESOURCES

FAVORITE BOOKS

Food Enzymes, Humbert Santillo, Hohm Press, Prescott Valley, Arizona

Fruit Can Heal You, Dr. Olm Abramouski, Nutritional and Natural Health Publications, P.O. Box 180, Westville, 3630, Natal, South Africa

How I Conquered Cancer Naturally, Eydie Mae with Chris Loeffler, Editorial Director, Harvest House Publishers, 1075 Arrowsmith, Eugene, Oregon 97407

Survival into the 21st Century, Viktorus Kulvinskas, Creation Publications, Distribution P.O. Box 702, Fairfield, Iowa 52556

Science of Breath, Yogi Ramacharaka, Yogi Publication Society, Chicago, IL, USA

Tissue Cleansing Through Bowel Management, Bernard Jensen, Route 1, Box 52, Escondido, CA 92025

Blatant Raw Foodist Propaganda, Joe Alexander, Blue Dolphin Publishing, Inc., P.O. Box 1908, Nevada City, CA 95959

Pottenger's Cats, Francis M. Pottenger, Jr., Price-Pottenger Nutrition Foundation, P.O. Box 2614, LaMesa, CA 92041 (619)582-4168

The End of Disease, David H. Fostiggi, World Congress for Peace Through Health, Inc., One Penn Plaza, Suite 100, New York, NY 10119

The Science and Fine Art of Fasting, Herbert M. Shelton, American National Hygiene Society, P.O. Box 30630, Tampa, Florida 33630

Enzyme Nutrition, Dr. Edward Howell, Avery Publishing Group, Inc., Wayne, New Jersey

Diet for a New America, John Robbins, Stillpoint Publishing, Box 640, Walpole, NH 03608

Fit for Life, Harvey Diamond

Light Eating for Survival, Marcia Madhuri Acciardo, 21st Century Publications, P.O. Box 702, Fairfield, Iowa 52536

The Uncook Book, Elizabeth & Dr. Elton Baker, Communication Creativity, P.O. Box 909, Buena Vista, CO 81211

Raw Energy, Leslie and Susannah Kenton, Arrow Books Limited, 62-65 Chandos Place, London WC2N 4NW, England

Laws of Success, Napoleon Hill, Success Unlimited, Inc., 1600 Orrington Avenue, Evanston, IL 60201

Spiritual Nutrition and The Rainbow Diet, Gabriel Cousens, MD, Cassandra Press, San Rafael, CA 94915

Live Food Juices, H. E. Kirschner, MD, H. E. Kirschner Publications, P.O. Box 36l, Monrovia, CA 91016

Own Your Own Body, Stan D. Malstrom, Keats Publishing Inc., New Canaan, CT

Is Menstruation Necessary, Wendy Harris, Nadine MacDonald

The Natural Way to Vibrant Health, Dr. N. W. Walker, Norwalk Press, 107 N. Cortez, Prescott, Arizona 86301

Roger's Recovery From AIDS, Bob Owen, Davar, P.O. Box 6310, Malibu, CA 90265

Why Suffer, Ann Wigmore, Avery Publishing Group, Inc., Wayne, New Jersey

AUDIO AND VIDEO TAPES

The Simple Power of Natural Herbs, Dean Black, Ph.D., Video, Tapestry Press, P.O. Box 563, Springville, VT 84663, (801) 489-7877

Angelic Harp Music, Erik Berglund c. 1988, Audio, Helios Enterprises (A MUST)

Diet for a New America, John Robbins, Video 1-800-765-7890,

60 minutes, KCET 4401 Sunset Blvd., Los Angeles, CA 90027

MAGAZINES

Health Science Magazine, American Natural Hygiene Society, P.O. Box 30630, Tampa, FL 33630

New Frontier Magazine, Magazine of Transformation, 101 Cuthbert St., Philadelphia, PA 19106 (215)627-5683

Index

Book Order Form

To obtain *Think Before You Eat*, mail orders to:

> **Diane Olive**
> **7536 Cowan Avenue**
> **Los Angeles, CA 90045**

For credit card orders, call (310) 645-9221

Please send me ___ softcover copies of *Think Before You Eat* at $12.95 + $2.00 for shipping and handling. _____

Subtotal $_____

Total $_____

Name:

_____

Address:

_____

City, State, Zip: _____

_____

Phone: _____

Artwork Order Form

To order 11 x 14 inch unframed color prints of art included in this book, mail order to:

Diane Olive
7536 Cowan Avenue
Los Angeles, CA 90045

For credit card orders, call (310) 645-9221

Artwork

Enter quantity wanted in front of each item

	Page	99	Listen from within	$65.00
___	Page	99	Listen from within	$65.00
___	Page	100	We all come from one	$65.00
___	Page	101	Little boxes	$65.00
___	Page	102/3	Aids man's teacher	$65.00
___	Page	104	The holy men *and*	
___	Page	105	Survival of the medical dark ages	$100.00
___	Page	106	Spin to become one *and*	
___	Page	106	Same painting spinning	$65.00
___	Page	107	Death in the four seasons	$65.00

Subtotal $_____

Shipping $ 2.00

(allow 4 to 6 weeks for processing & shipping)

Total $_____

Please send me ___ softcover copies of *Think Before You Eat* at $12.95 + $2.00 for shipping and handling.

Name:

_____

Address:

_____

City, State, Zip:_____

Phone: _____